Practising Clinical Supervision

A Reflective Approach

John Driscoll BSc(Hons), DPSN, Cert Ed, RNT, RMN, RGN
Formerly, Senior Lecturer, South Bank University, London, UK;
Unit Tutor, ENB RO1 (Clinical Supervision Skills for Supervisors)
Currently, Director: Transformational Learning Consultants Co Ltd

Forewords by
Professor Veronica Bishop
Department of Nursing and Midwifery,
De Montfort University Leicester,
Leicester, UK

Professor Tony Ghaye
Director of the Policy into Practice Research Centre,
University College Worcester,
Worcester, UK

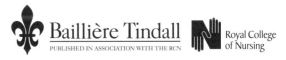

Baillière Tindall
PUBLISHED IN ASSOCIATION WITH THE RCN

Royal College
of Nursing

EDINBURGH LONDON NEW YORK PHILADELPHIA ST LOUIS SYDNEY TORONTO 2000

BAILLIÈRE TINDALL
An imprint of Harcourt Publishers Limited

© Harcourt Publishers Limited 2000

© Cartoons - Martin Davies

 is a registered trademark of Harcourt Publishers Limited

First published 2000

ISBN 0 7020 2419 8

British Library Cataloging in Publication Data
A catalogue record for this book is available from the British Library.

Library of Congress Cataloging in Publication Data
A catalog record for this book is available from the Library of Congress

Note
Medical knowledge is constantly changing. As new information becomes
available, changes in treatment, procedures, equipment and the use of drugs
become necessary. The author and the publishers have, as far as it is possible,
taken care to ensure that the information given in this text is accurate and
up-to-date. However, readers are strongly advised to confirm that the
information, especially with regard to drug usage, complies with the
latest legislation and standards of practice.

The
publisher's
policy is to use
**paper manufactured
from sustainable forests**

Printed in China

Contents

Forewords

The provision of health care has never been more complex, and the demands on health care professionals to forge multi-professional, multi-disciplinary and across-agency partnerships in the provision of that care are great. These demands cannot be met without two key constituents. Firstly, the ability of any health professional to understand and develop from peer review. Secondly, to be able to communicate, rather than just 'talk to' each other. Clinical supervision offers a framework that encourages, indeed, is central to these constituents. Implemented successfully, the evidence which is available indicates that a culture of caring critique, rather than a culture of blame, improves staff motivation. Integral to this process comes the opportunity for cross-fertilisation of skills, professional development and support, and communication skills – issues which are ignored at the peril of patient care.

The publication of this book is timely, and I congratulate the author on the production of such a practice-based addition to the growing body of literature on clinical supervision. This is meeting a genuine need, for while discussion has abounded on the subject and the UKCC has, since 1996, recommended its implementation, so have a plethora of misconceptions as to its functions. This has resulted in an apathy in some clinical localities in taking a vital mechanism forward for quality care. Some of the misconceptions derive from the term 'supervision', which has inappropriate connotations of a hierarchical system that must be anathema to a profession that is seeking to be autonomous. What is important about the terminology is that the focus is on clinical practice – the heart of what nursing is about – and it describes a mechanism to support the best in clinical developments (Bishop 1998). This very practical book builds on previous works by providing the reader with examples, or scenarios, on how to take clinical supervision forward.

Clinical supervision is about the professional entering into a relationship with clinical supervision itself, and having the confidence from that to enter into equal partnership with other health care professions. This is vital if nursing is to achieve its potential in making its contribution to health and health care. Changes and concomitant challenges sweep across the NHS with disconcerting speed. Boundaries between disciplines and agencies are becoming more and more blurred. Quite properly, patients and their carers are moving into the centre of health care focus, and nurses, perhaps more than any other group of health care professionals, are required to meet patients' needs in as flexible a manner as possible. Conceptually this is exciting, but the real world can sometimes appear to be beyond the scope of ideals, with the result that staff may be left feeling exhausted, distressed, out of touch and let down. The need to change a 'macho' style of management to one of caring critique is self-evident, particularly in the light of the dramatic current (and predicted) staff shortages suffered in the NHS. As Driscoll rightly states... 'there must be a genuine concern for the personal health of the workforce from within...'. I would also add that clinical supervision, if properly implemented, will be the greatest driver in taking forward excellence in care, and assure nursing's place at the clinical governance table.

The concept of clinical supervision is not 'yesterday's notion' – it is embedded in the recently published Department of Health document 'Making a Difference' (DoH 1999) and will be pivotal to nurses in taking forward the government's health care agenda. For this reason, management at every level must be committed to the success of clinical supervision. Clinical supervision is not a cheap option; it requires time, a budget, manpower and training. I fully agree with Driscoll that 'In the longer term, preparation... needs to become embedded in preregistration nurse education, where the continuum of clinical supervision really begins... In this way clinical supervision will be expected, as a continuation of lifelong learning.' (p. 80)

As I write this Foreword, on the eve of a new millennium, I am optimistic that with the benefit of such comprehensive and informative publications as this, the nursing profession, and any other which embraces the concept of clinical supervision, will achieve the maximum benefit from engaging in the process. Butterworth wrote that 'a future dream is to see any absence of clinical supervision as a curiosity; when that is so, we can be sure that its (integration) into the profession is complete.' This publication will, I am sure, make a significant contribution to achieving that reality.

Professor Veronica Bishop

REFERENCES

Bishop V 1998 Clinical supervision in Practice: some questions, answers and guidelines. Macmillan/NT Research, London
Butterworth A 1998 Clinical supervision in practice: some questions, answers and guidelines. Macmillan/NT Research, London
Department of Health 1999 'Making a Difference; strengthening the nursing, midwifery and health visiting contribution to health and health care. DoH, London
United Kingdom Central Council for Nursing, Midwifery and Health visiting 1996 Position Statement for Nursing and Health Visiting. London, UKCC

This is more than a good book - it is an excellent book and an essential read for all those who are, or plan to engage in clinical supervision. It is comprehensive and contains all the necessary information given the emerging quality agenda in healthcare. It is a practical book with lots of very well thought through ideas and actions that should help to make clinical supervision a meaningful lived reality for individuals and groups. Further, it is an exciting and challenging book. I am so pleased that John Driscoll has dared to address some of the more thorny and problematic aspects of both the nature and implementation of clinical supervision. To do this he has drawn upon an extensive and relevant literature and used his rich personal experience as a reflective healthcare practitioner. The publishers also need some credit for the way they have made the text accessible to the reader by the careful use of page layout, tables, figures and cartoons. I am sure you will enjoy this book and get much stimulation from it.

This book provides us with a framework for clinical supervision. In doing this it does not just value clinical supervision in its own right, so to speak, but argues passionately for its presence. Also it does not turn it into something 'soft', 'fluffy', 'warm' and 'cosy'. The message we get is that clinical supervision is about probing together, questioning practice, doubting, asking for help, enquiring. It is about taking a walk together into the whole field of human existence, beautifully captured by the reflective dimension of the text. Central to effective clinical supervision are 'relationships' and 'communication'. John Driscoll addresses these things. The style of the text invites the reader in, to participate in a process of learning and self/collective discovery. But he is careful not to tell us what to do, what to think, how we should behave and so on. So in this sense, this is also a book about freedom. Choice is not freedom. The book does not make us choose from the many conceptions of clinical supervision, from one list of skills or others. Choice in this sense is just moving in the same field, from one corner to another. The key to this freedom is expressed in chapter two, 'Reflective learning: the essence of clinical supervision'. Here John invites us to think again about our clinical work, to constructively challenge the status quo, to go further, to try to see practice more deeply and holistically. From this invitation he takes us on a journey which begins to come together when we get to chapter ten, 'From image to action: getting clinical supervision off the ground in the workplace'. It is at this point that we express our freedom. So what image/s do we have of clinical supervision? Which have we customised and for what reasons? What is/might work for us here? How do we think that this approach to clinical supervision might help us to enhance practice? How would we know this? It is at this point that the real complexity of moving from envisioning something to practising clinical supervision surfaces strongly. Clearly, John Driscoll wants us to appreciate that clinical supervision is not something easily defined and put into practice. It is a complex set of inter-relationships and interactions involving conscious and intentional healthcare professionals in technical, social, clinical and political acts-in-context. This is a book therefore that needs to be read more than once. This is partly due to the fact that it is a book of questions, tough, provocative and practice relevant questions. So in this sense it give us much to think about. It is not a quick read.

Above all else clinical supervision must be a learning process. Through its practise we should give ourselves an opportunity to learn more about what we do, why we do it this way and how the healthcare contexts in which we work serve to liberate or constrain us. Clinical supervision might best be seen as a process of becoming. This does not mean that through the process we always strive to reach conclusions and certainty, necessary though these are at times. Conclusions give us comfort, a sense of well-being and reassurance, a sense of stability and security. But clinical supervision can be more than this. John Driscoll helps us to appreciate that practising clinical supervision is also about releasing creative energy to bring about new or improved ways of seeing and doing. The book is about the creative energy of enquiry that enables us to penetrate practice, to investigate, explore, to open the door, to find out and to see further. This is the real essence of learning. This book gives us the courage to do just this.

Professor Tony Ghaye

Preface

The aim of this book is to provide an easy-to-read but thought-provoking practical guide to clinical supervision. It assumes no previous knowledge of clinical supervision and is intended for any healthcare practitioner but predominantly nurses, midwives and health visitors considering engaging in clinical supervision for the first time. It will be of use to newly qualified staff unfamiliar with the term clinical supervision, as well as more experienced staff who may think it has something to do with junior colleagues.

A simple definition of clinical supervision is 'formalised reflective practice in practice'. Unfortunately, that term 'reflective practice' will not seem to go away and, not unlike clinical supervision, is dependent on how committed you are in wanting to explore your clinical practice. This book will concern itself not with telling you how to do clinical supervision but with giving you the opportunity to reflect on how to get the most from engaging in the process. The emphasis of the book is towards the one-to-one encounter, while acknowledging that other forms of supervision exist and may be seen as more applicable in practice.

The text represents the start of a learning journey in clinical supervision, rather than a destination with a final endpoint. Many of you will have experienced how it is only after having finished a course of study that the real learning begins as you start to unravel some of the new ideas and transform new knowledge into the realities of your practice domain. Questioning what you have learned about clinical supervision and, more importantly, what you now intend to do with that new learning is a central theme of each chapter.

There will never be a single model of clinical supervision in practice, as the disciplines of nursing, midwifery, health visiting and healthcare practice are so diverse. Therefore, the development of clinical supervision in practice must be based on principles, with the actual process driven by practitioners according to the local situations in which they find themselves.

Clinical supervision is viewed by some authors as being introduced without the necessary evidence to support its implementation. Such arguments could also be laid at the door of reflective practice, yet such a process is now becoming a more familiar activity. My own view is that formalising clinical supervision is about organising regular time-out to critically reflect on, and obtain much-needed feedback about, aspects of your clinical practice – but in work time.

Often when practitioners are faced with controlling their own destiny in clinical practice, they need time to adjust to not having someone else telling them how to do it. Although the process can take longer, it is in this way that clinical supervision will become rooted in practice, because it is controlled and owned by people from within, not outside clinical practice. You are also charged with the responsibility of making more visible to others the value of engaging in clinical supervision, and identifying the links between clinical supervision and quality healthcare practice.

The development of clinical supervision knowledge is in its infancy in healthcare settings. It is my belief that the knowledge of how to do it is already embedded in everyday clinical practice, but has still to be fully identified and articulated. By regularly engaging in it, you will become part of the critical mass of healthcare practitioners in the 21st century who believe that a dynamic relationship exists between the provision of lifelong professional development and learning for clinicians and quality healthcare. Your personal experiences of doing so will, I hope, contribute to the development of specific knowledge about clinical supervision, in whichever healthcare environment you practise. Feel free to continue the supervision dialogue or comment on any aspect of this book and how it can be improved. Please write to: John Driscoll, Transformational Learning Consultants, Park Lodge, Waldingfield Road, Gallows Hill, Sudbury, Suffolk CO10 6QS, UK; e-mail address: johnd@ tlc-uk.com, website; http://www.tlc-uk.com

London 1999   John Driscoll

Acknowledgements

The fruition of this book concerns other people in my life who are excited, as well as not so excited, about the development of clinical supervision in healthcare practice. Perhaps least excited are my daughters Carly and Hayley, who once went on holiday, with my wife Anne and her parents Richard and Barbara, to facilitate my index-finger-tapping on the keyboard at home. I promise now to get on the end of the tea towel, regain my DIY prowess and find more time to spend together.

Reasonably excited are those I have been privileged to work with in clinical practice, who so readily shared their thoughts and ideas about workable schemes of clinical supervision and have influenced the content of the book. They include the practitioners and managers of BHB Community NHS Trust in Essex, specifically Corinne Hall, Debbie Sams, Hilary Shanahan, Paul Valoo, the 3-day retreat at London Colney with Helen Seijo, the original clinical supervisors' forum, and all course participants. Special mention must be made of: Forest NHS Trust in East London, specifically Heather Bartlett, Anne Connolly, Kathryn Robinson, Margaret Togher and all course participants; Redbridge Healthcare NHS Trust in Essex, specifically Paul Hanton, Jocelyn Hewitt, Mariola Lang, Maggie Lilley, Kim O'Connor, Gill Perry, Lynda Quinn, Sue Savage, the steering committee and all course participants; Havering Hospitals NHS Trust in Essex, specifically Gloria Dowling, Jacqui Harrison, Angela Keating, Miriam Lee, Rosemary Raeburn-Smith, the steering group and all course participants. I am also grateful to the social work practitioners on the ENB RO1 validation panel, particularly Margaret Poulter and Kip-Chan Pendsley but including a special thanks to Steve Cornish.

More than excited about the development of clinical supervision have been my long-suffering but supportive colleagues in the Faculty of Health, South Bank University. Special thanks must go to: Lesley Buckland for allowing me to immerse myself in clinical supervision while structural things were happening; Trudie James for her assistance in questionnaire design; John Kok, Kathy Nicholson, Ben Teh and Sue Williams for their support with the ENB RO1; my clinical supervisor Peter Davis and Professor Pam Smith for their invaluable publishing expertise; Chantal Thompson, Paula Hood and Diana Watmough in the library; and Catherine Heckman, my most ardent critic on the value of reflective practice in practice.

A significant influence has been Mic Rafferty at the University of Wales, for his support as an external adviser in the development of the ENB RO1, and for two cold and wet conference weekends in Swansea spent reflecting on ways the content of this book could be most helpful to clinical practitioners. I am also grateful to Chris Johns for his vision of transforming nursing through reflective practice, and all the participants at the Third Annual Conference on Reflective Practice, held at Robinson College, Cambridge in 1996, where this book was originally conceived.

Finally, special acknowledgement must go to Jacqueline Curthoys at Baillière Tindall for her own brand of guided reflection and supervision, which helped me to look towards blue skies when at times it was grey and lashing down.

How to get the most out of this book

There are two main premises of this book. The first is that clinical supervision is already happening in practice and has existed for many years. This book is about helping you recognise things that already go on in your practice that may mimic clinical supervision. If these things can be identified, it is likely that clinical supervision can be adapted into, rather than adopted for your clinical practice. Perhaps the most difficult thing to do is to regularly stop and review what has been going on, in what is often a hectic and complex delivery system within healthcare. Much of this book is not telling you what to do but intends being a source of help and support in getting clinical supervision off the ground in your practice area.

You may wish to simply dip in and out of the chapters, using some of the exercises or ideas to suit your needs rather than read it from cover to cover. Alternatively the way the book unrolls, allows you to again use some of the resources or ideas as a potential training programme for staff new to clinical supervision in your practice arena. Feel free to adapt or even photocopy the materials to meet your own needs.

The second premise of the book is to adopt a reflective approach to and in clinical supervision. This means more than just thinking about clinical supervision; it also means actioning some of that thinking. Throughout the chapters you will meet various icons that can help give you some direction or simply clarify what you have been reading. Some of them require you to stop and think of the implications of what you have been reading. Often it can be helpful to join up with a colleague or get some peer discussion going to get alternative views of what the icons ask you to do.

THINKING SPACE
This asks you to stop and think for a bit and consider the implications for yourself or your practice.

TIME OUT
This icon is often a doing exercise based on the material within the chapter which you can choose to do alone or with others in your practice area.

HAZARD WARNING
This icon is a warning that what is being described may not be as straightforward as it originally seemed!

HISTORY BOX

These are often personal descriptions or reflections based on the authors experiences of clinical supervision that serve to illustrate issues going on within the chapter. Often they are accompanied by a reflective dialogue or commentary to help clarify what is happening.

CARTOONS

Throughout the book are various cartoons that will serve as metaphors for what is actually trying to be conveyed. You might well still remember significant learning experiences for yourself because they seemed so stupid - and yet you can still remember them a long time after the learning event! Perhaps cartoons could form the basis of a learning journal or as reminders of significant events in practice or clinical supervision that might help in putting your own professional portfolio together. They certainly helped me in my own reflective writings in teacher training college! I still remember 'being bowled a googly' by a student sitting at the back of one of my first classes.

ON REFLECTION

At the end of each chapter appears a summary of the main content in the form of a structured model for reflection on practice which you can choose to do alone or with others in your practice area. You may feel that certain elements did not appear in the chapter summary. This book and clinical supervision will continually evolve with time. Contribute to the emerging knowledge of clinical supervision in practice by entering into further dialogue with the author based on what is happening in the book and what happens in your own practice domain (see Preface).

1 THE CONTEXT OF CLINICAL SUPERVISION

The purpose of Part 1 is to:

- broadly examine clinical supervision from a number of different perspectives and agendas other than for one's own clinical practice
- assist the reader to critically reflect on how the concept of clinical supervision may impact on their own practice domain
- empower the individual practitioner to consider and make choices about clinical supervision in the context of their own practice.

1 | What is clinical supervision?

INTRODUCTION

The contemporary nursing literature in general does not question the introduction of clinical supervision in practice. Perhaps this is because the Department of Health and the statutory bodies regulating nursing, midwifery and health visiting in the UK all suggest that clinical supervision in practice would be a 'good thing'. More probably, widespread implementation of the initiative has yet to happen, as practitioners struggle with what 'clinical supervision' actually means.

This first chapter intends to give an overview of what clinical supervision may or may not be. The reason for such apparent lack of clarity is that clinical supervision is only beginning to emerge alongside all the other activities that make up everyday clinical practice. Unlike other health-related disciplines, such as counselling or social work, where it is already established, the development of clinical supervision in nursing offers practitioners a unique opportunity to shape the form it should take in their own specialism.

To make informed decisions on how the process of clinical supervision can be incorporated into everyday nursing work, it is important to explore the background to its emergence and the different agendas and expectations that come with such an initiative. In facilitating workshops I have been interested to note how different clinical supervision appears when looked at from different points of view, for example those of a staff nurse who is wanting information on what is expected of them as a supervisee, of an assistant director of a community NHS healthcare trust who will be resourcing the initiative, or of a clinical manager seeking ways of managing such a change in clinical practice.

Whatever your perspective, for clinical supervision to be incorporated into everyday clinical practice it must have some demonstrable impact on the way nursing care is delivered. Although the ultimate challenge is for clinical supervision to equate to patient/client outcomes, initially a more obvious impact might be on the difference it makes to a practitioner and the way in which their work is subsequently carried out. An implicit assumption of clinical supervision is that regularly engaging in the process will enhance existing practice. In many respects, this will depend on what practitioners perceive such a process to be and more importantly why they should consider taking part in it.

SUPERVISION IN HEALTHCARE SETTINGS

The supervision of students by qualified nurses is a common event but the continued supervision of nurses, once qualified, is likely to be viewed as unusual. It is an interesting situation that for 3 years prior to qualifying as a nurse you are entitled to be given the necessary education and support to become an accountable practitioner, yet, once qualified and accountable inside the complex world of clinical practice, formalised supervision disappears after a rudimentary preparation period.

Although this is perhaps not quite true, because of the development of informal support mechanisms along the way and because it is possible to return for formal, supervised, courses of study, taking time out for yourself on a regular basis to obtain feedback on what you do is probably not the norm. Titchen & Binnie (1995) go further and suggest that, in adult nursing practice, supervision traditionally follows an 'industrial model of supervision', in which the production-line supervisor checks up on the workforce to spot omissions and errors rather than being concerned to facilitate the growth and development of the employee. Perhaps this model of supervision is also applicable to midwifery practice.

The statutory supervision of midwives has existed since the 1936 Midwives Act (Kirkham 1995) and is contained within Section 16 of the Nurses, Midwives and Health Visitors Act 1979 and outlined in Rules 44 and 45 of the *Midwife's Code of Practice* (UKCC 1994). Although the process is often promoted as offering guidance and direction to ensure that practice is correct, the supervisor of midwives is also able to formally discipline the midwife under supervision. The linking of clinical supervision to formal disciplinary processes is a continuing source of concern in midwifery practice (Seaman 1995).

While it may be tempting to simply 'borrow' supervision knowledge from other disciplines, it is also worth considering that you will have different needs and circumstances in your own specialist areas of practice. Although the UKCC continues to endorse the way midwifery supervision is organised, it states that the development of clinical supervision in nursing and health visiting is not a managerial control system, hierarchical in nature, nor a statutory requirement (UKCC 1996). That is why clinical supervision in nursing and health visiting is not an exact science (or ever likely to be), will take time to be developed from within practice by practitioners and will not be successful if it is thrust on practitioners by those outside.

In other health-related disciplines, regular feedback on clinical practice for qualified practitioners is not an unusual feature. Not surprisingly, the nursing literature on the development of clinical supervision has become interested in disciplines where supervision is already an integral part of clinical practice, such as social work (Davies 1988, Kadushin 1992, Pritchard 1995, Brown & Bourne 1996, Morrison 1996), counselling and psychotherapy (Westheimer 1977, Casement 1985, Houston 1990, Hawkins & Shohet 1992, Holloway 1995, Hughes & Pengelly 1997).

Because of the historical development of clinical supervision within psychotherapy, counselling and social work, the concept is not unfamiliar to mental health nurses. Although not yet the norm for the majority of mental health nurses (Carson et al 1995, p. 54), it is another opportunity for nurses to explore (and share with others in steering groups) what elements of supervision could be valuable in nursing practice. In some cases this might include potentially being supervised by those who already have expertise in supervision but are not necessarily nurses. Looking at other disciplines can clarify the range of supervision possibilities for nursing practice. Swain, discussing clinical supervision in health visiting, begins by stating what clinical supervision is *not* before elaborating on what it is: 'Clinical supervision is not psychotherapy or counselling. This must be clearly understood. Nor is it directive management, individual performance review …, or staff appraisal. It is not a form of disciplinary procedure … or any of those many things which some nurses seem to fear it might be or could be used for' (Swain 1995, p. 16).

Once again, beware of blindly adopting other people's models of supervision into your own area of practice simply because they are in close proximity or have a structural relationship with your practice.

Read Swain's (1995) statement again.
If clinical supervision in nursing and health visiting is not counselling or psychotherapy, nor a mandatory managerial imposition, what then is it likely to be?

Timpson (1996) in a substantial review of the literature on clinical supervision in relation to cancer nursing, cites Hawkins & Shohet's (1992) analogy of supervision as being 'pit head' time, whereby: 'practitioners are able to "wash off" all the emotional grime and detritus of the day in works time, much as miners cleanse themselves of coal dust which permeates every part of their being, before going home'.

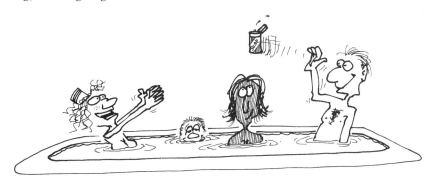

This gives a potential focus for clinical supervision in nursing practice that is not counselling, psychotherapy or imposed by clinical managers. It is also a challenging proposition for managers to arrange time during work for practitioners to reflect on what is happening, or has happened, with others in order to survive the physical and psychological demands of caring. It is interesting to compare the 'pit head time' analogy with the different ways clinical supervision is more formally defined within the nursing literature.

DEFINING CLINICAL SUPERVISION

Although this text assumes no previous knowledge, it would be very surprising if you could not, from prior experience, imagine what 'clinical supervision' might be in practice from the two words alone.

Clinical

supervision

Many of your thoughts will, I suspect, be strongly influenced by your own positive and not so positive experiences of being 'supervised' in clinical practice. Your past experiences may even influence whether or not you get involved in the clinical supervision initiative. Fish & Twinn (1997, p. 16) remind us that forms of supervision have been around in nursing for some time: these have already been touched upon. They usefully differentiate between two different modes of clinical supervision, which are developed in more detail in a later chapter, 'the on course mode, where the supervisor operates within the context of a professionally focused course, and the professional development mode where the supervisor works with a qualified practitioner in the context of their daily work'.

This not only covers preregistration students requiring supervision to develop expertise, but also introduces the theme of the continual professional development of an already qualified practitioner not necessarily involved in any formal study. Clinical supervision is linked to the maintenance of professional registration by offering an alternative route to individual professional development (UKCC 1997, p. 11). It also indicates that, even if you have been on a study course recently, there is still no 'endpoint' of maintaining and developing standards of practice. The UKCC (1996) continues this theme by stating that clinical supervision 'will assist lifelong learning by being accessible to all registered practitioners throughout their careers'.

How many qualified practitioners reading this might consider starting their shift as a learner in practice by stating:
'What I intend to learn in practice today is...'
or, after the shift has finished, telling themselves:
'What I learned in practice today was...'

More probably, any opportunities for reflective learning in practice, such as a handover period or completion of the documentation of a patient/client at the end of a shift, will normally be confined to a description of what was done or has happened. This is discussed in more detail in the next chapter. Talking to each other about practice, in practice, features in probably the most widely quoted definition of clinical supervision in the nursing literature, that offered by Butterworth:

> Clinical supervision is an exchange between practising professionals to enable the development of professional skills (Butterworth 1992, p. 12).

The need to formalise talking to one another during work time in order to learn, as well as to support each other in practice, is legitimised by the chief nursing officers of the UK. *A Vision for the Future* (Department of Health 1993), in seeking to provide a blueprint for nursing, midwifery and health visiting into the new millennium, emphasised the development of clinical supervision as one of the key elements enabling registered nurses to maintain clinical competence and be more personally responsible for their own practice. It is described as:

> a term used to describe a formal process of professional support and learning which enables individual practitioners to develop knowledge and competence, assume responsibility for their own practice and enhance consumer protection and safety of care in complex situations (Department of Health 1993).

Subsequently, the chief nursing officer for England, Yvonne Moores, stated her own belief in clinical supervision in an accompanying letter (Department of Health 1994): 'I have no doubt as to the value of Clinical Supervision and consider it to be fundamental to safeguarding standards, the development of professional expertise and the delivery of quality care'.

Both the previous definitions, not surprisingly, offer the 'what' of clinical supervision. Kohner's definition begins to offer the 'how':

> Clinical supervision is a formal arrangement enabling nurses to discuss their work regularly with another experienced professional. It involves reflecting on practice in order to learn from experience and improve competence (Kohner 1994).

Bishop offers an equally pragmatic definition as a baseline for the realities of clinical practice:

> Clinical supervision is a designated interaction between two or more practitioners, within a safe/supportive environment, which enables a continuum of reflective, critical analysis of care, to ensure quality patient services (Bishop 1998, p. 8).

To happen in practice, clinical supervision is reliant on supportive management, for whom the concept can have a more managerial connotation. McCallion & Baxter (1995) adapted Worsley's (1994) definition for implementation in practice. The background of the authors in management and education is reflected in a different type of emphasis:

> Supervision is a mandatory or negotiated contractual relationship between a supervisor and supervisee in which the worker gives an account of his/her work with the express purpose of developing their competence in providing the highest quality of service to the client or customer (McCallion & Baxter 1995).

Finally, the conclusions of Professor Chris Maggs (1994), in a substantive work trying to pin down the elusive concept of 'mentor', could be borrowed for the similarly elusive concept of clinical supervision – that, although there is confusion about what it is, it seems to be regarded as a way of helping individuals develop their professional practice!

The thing to remember is that clinical supervision is not an exact science and, while the term itself could be a barrier to implementation, practitioners need to establish ownership of the process by developing their own working definition of it. As Butterworth (1998, p. 11) reminds us, clinical supervision is not, and should never be, yet another imposition placed on those in clinical practice by management or academics.

A true definition of clinical supervision is still up for grabs, as practitioners in different areas wrestle with the principles that underpin it, and attempt to incorporate it in clinical practice. The one you settle on may be a hybrid of others, the same one as someone else, or a completely new one. What is essential is that, as a group of practitioners, you first discuss the range of options and then agree on what the term means to you. This important element of the implementation of clinical supervision is discussed in more detail in Chapter 10.

Looking again at the different definitions of clinical supervision, what key phrases or words seem to recur, suggesting that they are significant components of clinical supervision?
Compare your own ideas to the summary contained in Box 1.1

BOX 1.1	Key phrases in definitions of clinical supervision

- a formal process of professional support and learning
- assuming responsibility for practice
- enabling practitioners to share and learn from experience
- enhancing consumer protection and safety of care
- a formal arrangement enabling nurses to discuss their work
- regularly learning from experience and improving competence
- sustaining and developing professional practice
- the development of professional skills
- reflective practice
- quality patient services
- a designated time for interaction between practitioners

SOME WORKING ASSUMPTIONS ABOUT CLINICAL SUPERVISION

Many of the words you probably identified in the definitions relate to issues involving continuing professional development and the need for support in an ever-changing healthcare landscape. Butterworth (1998, p. 13), in his position statement for both mentorship and clinical supervision, identifies a number of ground rules for nursing practice:

- Skills should be constantly redefined and improved throughout professional life
- Critical debate about practice activity is a means to professional development
- Clinical supervision offers protection to independent and accountable practitioners

- Introduction to a process of clinical supervision should begin in professional training and education, and continue thereafter as an integral part of professional development
- Clinical supervision requires time and energy and is not an incidental event.

These points can also be viewed as a philosophy, embodying a number of values for any practice area thinking about starting clinical supervision. As with any philosophy in practice, it should be modified by your own values and beliefs and, like the ground rules for clinical supervision, will change and need to be amended over time.

Probably one of the most challenging of the rules, and one that is dealt with in a later chapter, is the need to find the time for clinical supervision among all the other time pressures facing you in practice. This will require commitment to the initiative, and regarding clinical supervision as 'sacred space' to give back to yourself instead of constantly giving your time to others. It may involve temporarily not being available to others by physically removing yourself into your agreed 'sacred space' off the clinical area. Obviously, the commitment to clinical supervision does not in practice extend only to yourself but is dependent on your colleagues and, importantly, on your manager legitimising the use of the time.

It is interesting to note that the ground rules appear to have stood the test of time since they were originally published in 1992, and that they mesh very well with the reasons why clinical supervision has emerged and continues to remain high on the political and professional agendas to carry nursing into a new millennium. While definitions are often the stated ideals of something, to find out what the reasons for implementing clinical supervision are it is worth exploring the background to how it emerged in the first place.

THE EMERGENCE OF CLINICAL SUPERVISION IN NURSING PRACTICE

Much of the drive towards introducing clinical supervision derived from the rapid changes in healthcare delivery and the response to these of the nurses who had to adapt to them. The changes can be broadly categorised as:

- political
- professional
- managerial
- ethicolegal
- educational
- personal.

Taken as a whole they represent some of the reasons for implementing clinical supervision and are summarised in Figure 1.1.

You can probably think of some other factors in addition to those listed. You may have been surprised by how much impetus is behind the implementation of the initiative. Clinical supervision has recently been given added impetus by governmental proposals for radical and far reaching quality reforms in the NHS under the umbrella of clinical governance (Department of Health 1997, 1998a, 1998b).

Figure 1.1   *Factors influencing the emergence of clinical supervision in practice*

Political
- More health care being carried out in the community
- More acute care needed for patients staying in hospital
- Nurses, Midwives and Health Visitors Act 1979 under review
- Support for clinical supervision by chief nursing officers of the UK
- Increased individual responsibility and accountability in clinical care
- Numerous reviews/reports recommend uptake of clinical supervision
- The 'Beverley Allitt affair'
- Reduced central function and increased autonomy of local systems of healthcare
- Increased emphasis on clinical effectiveness in care delivery (clinical governance)
- Development of an increasingly outcomes orientated NHS
- The setting of national standards in healthcare
- Devolved responsibility and accountability for care (clinical governance)
- Promotion of links between continued professional development of staff and quality of care (clinical governance)

Professional
- Increased scope/accountability in professional practice with the reduction in junior doctors' hours
- Increased personal responsibility and accountability of the individual practitioner
- Adoption of a more individual approach to care
- Acknowledgement that nursing is stressful and requires active support in practice
- Acceptance that empowerment strategies for patients can also be of value to staff
- Promotion of the therapeutic use of self in nursing
- Maintenance of registration through self regulation activities
- Reports and reviews on practice supporting the development of clinical supervision
- Support for specialist nurse led initiatives
- Support for network activities and multidisciplinary working
- The development of clinical leadership schemes in practice

Personal

Managerial
- Flattening of traditional hierarchies in nursing practice
- More open approach to sharing what goes on in neighbouring organisations
- Difficulties in recruiting and retaining qualified staff in practice
- Expanded practice development activities
- Increased support for innovations as team building activities
- Recognition of increased staff isolation in primary care
- More formalised collaboration with medical and allied staff
- Emphasis on more effective use of resources including human ones
- Development of clinical effectiveness activities
- Increased amount of staff led innovation in practice
- Recognition of the need for formalised support systems to lessen burn out and work related stress
- Concerns about the implications and necessary role preparation for clinical governance
- Increased emphasis on effectively managing risk
- Implications of the Beverley Allitt affair
- More emphasis on setting standards and patient outcomes
- Increased level of formal patient complaints about practice
- Demarcation of individual responsibilities associated with anticipated care pathways
- Increased use of measurement in relation to practitioner activities
- Concerns about promoting the health of the workforce
- Reductions in annual insurance premiums for organisations proactively managing risk

Ethicolegal
- Difficult choices in allocating scarce resources and effect on staff welfare
- Patient now a more knowledgeable consumer of healthcare with rights
- Active promotion of patients' rights in healthcare
- Increased incidence of complaints by health users and potential litigation
- Reduction in junior doctors' hours and increased responsibility/accountability of practitioners
- Increased need to monitor autonomous staff
- More awareness by staff of ethicolegal implications of caring and associated staff dilemmas and stress at work
- Increased emphasis on reducing costs with an expanding workload and associated risks to individuals and the organisation
- Increased media focus on poor aspects of organisational healthcare delivery
- Increased use of 'naming and blaming' in healthcare and associated penalties
- Increased use of legal services by organisations to advise on practice
- Increased anxiety associated with the development of clinical governance frameworks to ensure quality of care

Educational
- Development of practice based evidence initiatives as well as evidence based practice courses
- Increased demand by practitioners for development of specialist, rather than 'borrowed' knowledge for practice
- Unsupported practitioners in practice unable to support effective learning in practice
- Increased collaborative networking and sharing that learning with practice
- Collaborative development of continuing professional development strategies to support quality care initiatives in practice
- An increased association by practitioners that developing reflective strategies in practice can help support innovation in practice
- Increased emphasis by qualified practitioners to learn communication and interpersonal techniques for use in practice
- Increased development of informal learning strategies in practice that can contribute to practitioner PREP requirements and lifelong learning, e.g. AP(E)L, maintaining portfolios, learning journals, and clinical supervision
- Increased demand to develop a range of clinical supervision courses tailored to suit organisational needs
- Increased demand for research expertise alongside organisation implementation of clinical supervision
- Emphasis on devolving responsibility for practitioners to develop models of clinical supervision from within practice

As will be seen in later chapters, many of these reforms dovetail neatly into ideas about what clinical supervision aims to achieve in practice. More detailed accounts of the development of clinical supervision can be found in Fowler 1996, Bond & Holland 1998, Dolley et al 1998 (p. 141), and Brocklehurst 1999.

The personal reasons for a practitioner to engage in clinical supervision have been left out. This does not mean that they are not important: it is to remind you that you must make them known to others. Working as you do in health-care, you have played an indirect part in the collective reasons listed for the development of clinical supervision in practice.

How much do you agree personally with the influencing factors behind the emergence of clinical supervision? Do they appear simply to come from the top down or do you think they actually reflect aspects of your own learning, responsibilities and support mechanisms in practice?

Your initial response to clinical supervision could be a bit cynical when you consider your past experiences and the length of time you have spent in health-care. Perhaps your own experience of any new development in practice is that you are often the last to be consulted, if at all, and then, all of a sudden, it's happening. Not clinical supervision, however. Quite simply, it cannot be developed without the individual support and commitment of practitioners.

If you do not feel that you own part of the development of clinical super-vision – and why should you at this stage? – will you be likely to cover a colleague or a new staff member wishing to 'pop next door' for an hour's clinical supervision, or vice versa? This is one example of how proceeding with clinical supervision requires the support of everybody concerned – perhaps even your group of patients! One of the ways to feel involved is to consider your own personal agenda in clinical supervision as well as everybody else's.

DISCOVERING YOUR OWN AGENDA IN CLINICAL SUPERVISION

Looking back over what has been discussed in this chapter, the emphasis has largely been on identifying what clinical supervision may or may not be, accord-ing to other people who think they know about you and your practice. The push towards the implementation of clinical supervision is also driven by concerns arising from structural changes in health provision, education and clinical prac-tice and an overdue recognition of the stressful nature of nursing itself. In what ways are other people's agendas for implementing clinical supervision similar to or different from your own, and what might be the consequences of that?

Compare your own thoughts about clinical supervision as an individual practitioner to some expressed in introductory workshops on clinical supervision (Box 1.2).

How do these relate to your own ideas?

BOX 1.2	*Some contrasting images of clinical supervision expressed in introductory workshops*

- Time out for **me** in work time where I am the focus of attention
- Dedicated time to reflect on **my** practice
- A mechanism for facilitating **my** personal and professional development
- A source of professional support for **me** during new or difficult practice situations
- An opportunity to explore **my** clinical practice in a safe environment and learn from **my** practice experiences

- Something obligatory imposed by management on all clinical practitioners
- A requirement from my professional organisation(s)
- A surveillance or monitoring tool for me by management
- Another idea from those outside practice for those inside practice
- It won't work because there's not enough time during the shift now
- We're doing it already anyway
- We support one another already without needing to formalise it

BOX 1.3	*Expectations of clinical supervision*

Organisational

- Improvement or maintenance of practice standards
- A professional support mechanism in practice by practice
- Possible reductions in sickness and absenteeism
- A mechanism for ensuring safe practice
- Increased recruitment and retention of staff
- Reduction in complaints about clinical practice
- Support for innovation in practice
- Increased team spirit and morale
- Noticeable changes in the performance of practitioners in clinical supervision
- More critical questioning and generation of solutions to practice problems

Practitioners

- A formalised source of support in practice
- Reduced stress by being given time to formally explore any source of stress with others
- An opportunity to seek new ways to be more in control of practice
- Reflection on practice offers a learning dimension to just 'doing the work'
- Increased self-awareness of how practice is being delivered
- An alternative way of maintaining professional registration and fulfilling PREP requirements
- Promotes motivation to explore practice issues more deeply

BOX 1.3 cont.	*Expectations of clinical supervision*

- Helps to develop self-confidence and job satisfaction
- Assists with adapting to changes in practice

Patients (speculative only)

- Seems to be confident when looking after me?
- Seems to be knowledgeable about my condition?
- Seems to be interested in my experience of healthcare?
- Seems to be using me to learn more about my condition and circumstances?
- Seems to 'go the extra mile' with people in his/her care?
- Seems to have an open and honest approach when looking after me?
- Seems to know where he/she is going as a nurse?

It would seem that a lot of different people have a stake in the successful implementation of clinical supervision (Box 1.3).

Perhaps the biggest danger to warn against is the high expectations that everybody has about what clinical supervision is supposed to do in practice. While there is undoubtedly much support for clinical supervision from 'on high', it will not be given to practitioners on a plate (Dolley et al 1998, p. 142). I am reminded of an early warning in the literature issued by Bishop (1994): 'While clinical supervision will help nurses to achieve the best level of care possible, it cannot compensate for inadequate facilities, for poor management or for unmotivated staff. However it will create a culture within which nurses can flourish if they are willing to embrace it and if management is supportive.'

On reflection ... chapter summary

Being more aware of the different agendas that exist about clinical supervision will help in addressing the enormous task of rooting clinical supervision firmly within practice. It will not happen overnight. Much will depend on the experience and ongoing relationship of the supervisor and supervisee. Effective clinical supervision involves not only the skills of the clinical supervisor but also the development of supervisory skills by the supervisee. Both these elements are covered in detail in later chapters.

This chapter has endeavoured to give you a chance to think about clinical supervision and has probably supplied more questions than answers. While not all reflective practice is clinical supervision, all clinical supervision is reflective practice. Indeed, clinical supervision could be more simply defined as formalised reflective practice in practice (Driscoll 1996), which is the subject of the next chapter.

REFERENCES

Bishop V 1994 Clinical supervision for an accountable profession. Nursing Times 90(39): 35–37

Bishop V (ed) 1998 Clinical supervision in practice: some questions, answers and guidelines. Macmillan/Nursing Times Research Publications, London

Bond M, Holland S 1998 Skills of clinical supervision for nurses. Open University Press, Buckingham

Brocklehurst N, Walshe K 1999 Quality and the new NHS. Nursing Standard 13 (15) 46–53

Brown A, Bourne I 1996 The social work supervisor. Open University Press, Milton Keynes

Butterworth T 1992 Clinical supervision as an emerging idea in nursing. In: Butterworth T, Faugier J (eds) Clinical supervision and mentorship in nursing. Chapman & Hall, London, p 3–17

Butterworth T 1998 Clinical supervision as an emerging idea in nursing. In: Butterworth T, Faugier J, Burnard P (eds) Clinical supervision and mentorship in nursing, 2nd edn. Stanley Thornes, Cheltenham, p 1–18

Carson J, Fagin L, Ritter SA 1995 Stress and coping in mental health nursing. Chapman & Hall, London

Casement P 1985 On learning from the patient. Routledge, London

Davies M 1988 Supervision models. In: Staff supervision in the probation service. Avebury, Aldershot, ch 5, p 113–141

Department of Health 1993 Vision for the future: the nursing, midwifery and health visiting contribution to health and health care. HMSO, London

Department of Health 1994 Clinical supervision for the nursing and health visiting professions. CNO Letter 94 (5). HMSO, London

Department of Health 1997 NHS white paper - the new NHS, modern, dependable. Department of Health, London

Department of Health 1998a A first class service - quality in the new NHS. Department of Health, London

Department of Health 1998b Working together - securing a quality workforce for the NHS. Department of Health, London

Dolley J, Davies C, Murray P 1998 Clinical supervision: a development pack for nurses (K509). Open University Press, Buckingham

Driscoll JJ 1996 Reflection and the management of community nursing. British Journal of Community Health Nursing 1(2): 92–96

Fish D, Twinn S 1997 Quality clinical supervision in the health care professions: principled approaches to practice. Butterworth-Heinemann, London

Fowler J 1996 The organisation of clinical supervision within the nursing profession: a review of the literature. Journal of Advanced Nursing 23: 471–478

Hawkins P, Shohet R 1992 Supervision in the helping professions. Open University Press, Milton Keynes

Holloway EL 1995 Clinical supervision: a systems approach. Sage, London

Houston G 1990 Supervision and counselling. Rochester Foundation, London

Hughes L, Pengelly P 1997 Staff supervision in a turbulent environment: managing process and task in front-line services. Jessica Kingsley, London

Kadushin A 1992 Supervision in social work, 3rd edn. Columbia University Press, New York

Kirkham M 1995 The history of midwifery supervision. In: Association of Radical Midwives (ed) Super-vision: consensus conference proceedings. Books For Midwives Press, Hale

Kohner N 1994 Clinical supervision in practice. King's Fund Centre, London

McCallion H, Baxter T 1995 Clinical supervision: how it works in the real world. Nursing Management 1(9): 20–21

Maggs C 1994 Mentorship in nursing and midwifery education: issues for research. Nurse Education Today 14: 22–29

Morrison T 1996 Staff supervision in social care. Pavilion, Brighton

Pritchard J (ed) 1995 Good practice in supervision: statutory and voluntary organisations. Jessica Kingsley, London

Seaman B 1995 Where supervision goes wrong. In: Association of Radical Midwives (ed) Super-vision: consensus conference proceedings. Books For Midwives Press, Hale

Swain G 1995 Clinical supervision: the principles and process. Health Visitors Association, London

Timpson J 1996 Clinical supervision: a plea for 'pit head time' in cancer nursing. European Journal of Cancer Care 5: 43–52

Titchen A, Binnie A 1995 The art of clinical supervision. Journal of Clinical Nursing 4: 327–334

UKCC 1994 The Midwife's Code of Practice. United Kingdom Central Council for Nursing, Midwifery and Health Visiting, London

UKCC 1996 Position statement on clinical supervision for nursing and health visiting. United Kingdom Central Council for Nursing, Midwifery and Health Visiting, London

UKCC 1997 PREP and you. United Kingdom Central Council for Nursing, Midwifery and Health Visiting, London

Westheimer I 1977 The practice of supervision in social work: a guide for supervisors. Ward Lock Educational, London

Worsley P 1994 Supervision. Organisational and Personal Development Consultants (OPDC), Somerset

FURTHER READING

Butterworth T, Carson J, White E, Jeacock A, Clements A, Bishop V 1997 It is good to talk. An evaluation study in England and Scotland. The School of Nursing, Midwifery and Health Visiting, University of Manchester, Manchester, UK

Collaborative Clinical Supervision Project 1999 (in association with North Warwickshire NHS Trust) Clinical Super...Vision Open Learning Pack. Birmingham, UK

Department of Health 1994 The Allitt Inquiry. Independent Inquiry Relating to Deaths and Injuries on the Children's Ward at Grantham and Kesteven General Hospital during the Period February to April 1991. Clothier Report, HMSO, London, UK

English National Board 1995 Creating Life-Long Learners - Partnerships for Care, ENB, London, UK

Fatchett A 1998 Nursing in the new NHS: Modern, Dependable? Balliere-Tindall, London, UK

Faugier J, Butterworth T 1994 Clinical Supervision: A Position Paper (given at the first Department of Health Conference on Clinical Supervision in Birmingham). School of Nursing Studies, University of Manchester: 1-60

Gadd D, Manhood N 1995 Clinical Supervision: A Time for Professional Development on Internet website: http://tin.ssc.plym.ac.uk/cartmel/clinsup2.html, University of Plymouth, Plymouth, UK

Lillyman S, Ghaye T 2000 Effective clinical supervision: The role of reflection. Quay books, Mark Allen Publishing, Salisbury, UK

National Health Service Executive 1996 Clinical supervision- a resource pack for practice nurses. NHSE, London, UK

National Health Service Executive 1995 Clinical Supervision- A Resource Pack for London Practice Nurses. NHSE, London, UK

The Open University 1998 Clinical Supervision: A Development Pack for Nurses (K509) The Open University School of Health and Social Welfare, Open University Press, Milton Keynes, UK

Royal College of Nursing Institute 1999 Realising Clinical Effectiveness and Clinical Governance through Clinical Supervision: A Distance Learning Pack. Radcliffe Medical Press, Oxon, UK

RCN 1998 Nursing Update Video (Learning Unit 077) Caring together: clinical supervision broadcast by the BBC2 Learning Zone on 26 February and 5 March by Marrow C, Yaseen T, Cook M and featured in Nursing Standard 12(22): 1-27

Wallace M 1999 Lifelong Learning PREP in Action. Churchill Livingstone, Edinburgh , UK

West Midlands Clinical Supervision Learning Set 1998 Clinical Supervision: Getting it right in your organisation A critical guide to good practice. West Midlands Clinical Supervision Learning Set, c/o School of Health Sciences, University of Birmingham, Birmingham, UK

Reflective learning: the essence of clinical supervision?

INTRODUCTION

This chapter highlights what could be argued is the essence of clinical supervision – reflective practice. While not all reflective practice is clinical supervision, all clinical supervision is based on being reflective about practice. Many practitioners believe that they are already reflective in practice (Reid 1993) and so, perhaps rightly, question why they need clinical supervision. What they probably mean is that in their daily work they are constantly having to think about what they are doing. But reflection and particularly reflective learning is more than just thinking about something.

The previous chapter examined the expectations for practitioners engaging in clinical supervision and how it is intended to help bring about changes in practice. Johns & Freshwater (1998) believe that it is possible to transform nursing through reflective practice. Lumby (1998, p. 91) asserts that, unless being reflective in practice is manifested in some form of action, it is not transformation but something else.

Clinical supervision does give practitioners a legitimate opportunity to regularly stop and think, in the midst of practice, with the intention of enhancing what already happens in that practice. If actions occur by a supervisee as a result of talking to the clinical supervisor, then clinical supervision through reflective learning may well be able to transform whole areas of practice.

This chapter will help you gain more understanding of what reflection is and consider whether you are already engaging in the process of reflective learning. Gaining an insight into reflective learning will:

- help you become more self-aware in your clinical practice
- help you discover, rather than passively read someone else's ideas about, clinical supervision in practice

■ decide whether reflective learning as the essence of clinical supervision has the potential to transform your clinical practice.

HOW REFLECTION IS MORE THAN JUST THINKING

Jarvis (1992) suggested that no profession has reflective practice; however professionals do have the ability to practice reflectively, though this does not mean they will reflect, only that the potential to do so exists within them. Clinical supervision offers such a potential, by the legitimisation of regular time-out to discuss significant practice issues with the help of a clinical supervisor. Effective clinical supervision is more than having a chat with a colleague over a cup of coffee.

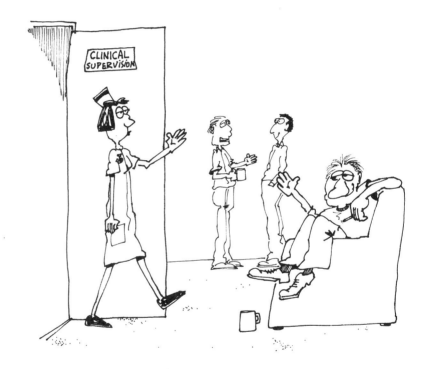

Although an important activity in which to help recover from the stresses and strains of nursing practice, clinical supervision requires commitment and motivation to reflect on practice regularly and is more than just thinking. It is important to differentiate thinking and reflection as two different activities. This will also challenge the assumption that you are already doing it ... but doing what?

Jane is the manager of Hillside Nursing Home. Read in sequence the accounts contained in the History Box, and the commentary below on what is happening. You should be able to begin to differentiate between Jane thinking and Jane being reflective.

History Box

Monday

On Monday, while driving to the nursing home, Jane is thinking 'Where did I put that phone number for getting some flowers delivered to Mum for her birthday on Wednesday?... Ooh! I must nip out at lunchtime to get some tea and coffee, as we'll need that in the morning.... It's going to be desperate this week with John on annual leave, I only hope that Anne doesn't go off sick, as I'm supposed to be going on a clinical supervision workshop on Wednesday ... or was it Thursday?.... I must remember to do the off duty, it's supposed to be in the diary by tomorrow.... Am I going to make the lights?... *Hurry up over, you idiot!*... Phew, that was close!'

Commentary

In this example lots of images and thoughts appear to be racing around in Jane's mind during her drive to work. Although seemingly pressing concerns, they could be considered aimless, as very little real thought appears to be going on about how Jane can resolve her difficulties. Which one is the main priority? If Jane was asked an hour later to remember what those thoughts were, I wonder whether she would have forgotten and replaced them with something else? Perhaps the main priority – actually getting to work safely in the car – has somehow been overlooked!

Wednesday

On Wednesday, Jane has popped into to see her Mum on the way to the clinical supervision workshop at the local university college, but has not anticipated the amount of school traffic at that time of the morning. She turns up 10 minutes late, in a bit of a panic; suddenly she realises that the background reading she was asked to do prior to the workshop has been left on top of the fridge since last week.

Later, as one of the senior staff members in attendance, Jane is asked by the lecturer, 'What opportunities exist for reflection in your nursing home?' She thinks to herself, 'Why did he pick on me? I can't remember what reflection is ... it's a long time since I've done any studying.... What's the point of clinical supervision anyway? We won't have any time for it.' Jane becomes flustered, thinking to herself, 'What must other people in the group think of me?... Perhaps I can bluff my way out.... The proprietor of Hillside will be expecting me to take back some idea of what clinical supervision is about ... I'm supposed to be the lead for it.'

Jane then blurts out to the group 'The best time I find to do reflection is when we are handing over shifts!'

Commentary

In this example, an unanticipated event leads to Jane's late attendance and a sudden realisation that the background reading has not been done. This is compounded by Jane becoming aware of the centrality of her role in implementing clinical supervision in the nursing home. There does seem to be some evidence of more active and reasoned thinking by Jane, in response to the question posed by the lecturer, than what she was doing in the car on Monday.

However, the limited time Jane has to answer, and her awkward feelings about not having done anything previously and not wanting to look stupid, create a barrier that gets in the way of fully answering the question. Jane is able to rely on her previous experience of clinical practice in the nursing home and manages to conjure up a 'reactive' answer to pacify the lecturer in class. Some of the uncomfortable feelings Jane has experienced, lead to actions 2 days later.

Friday

On Friday evening, Jane is having a quiet cup of coffee in the kitchen while everyone else in the family is watching television. It's been a bad week. She begins to replay in her mind what significant things have happened to her that week. The flowers she had organised Monday lunchtime didn't arrive until the day after her Mum's birthday, as the florist had taken down the wrong house number and they were delivered further up the street.

It seemed that, after arriving late at the college, things went from bad to worse. Jane thinks to herself, 'Apart from the lecturer picking on me ... probably because I was late ... he asked me afterwards if I would like to participate in a joint clinical supervision project for the nursing home ... well, actually it's not really a project, he just suggested it would be a good idea to first canvass staff reactions to clinical supervision.... The trouble is with being understaffed and people always going off sick, I already have enough on my plate ... mind you, if we could establish some regular time out for ourselves as a staff group we could perhaps begin to look after one another a bit more than we do now ... it might even help the sickness rates!

'I must try to organise my time better and adopt a more helpful attitude with the junior staff. I'll see Julie, the deputy manager, on Monday.... I seem to remember her talking to me about the course she is doing that involves her looking at time management. If the lecturer wants me to find out more from the staff about clinical supervision ... perhaps he will help me devise a questionnaire.'

Commentary

This final example demonstrates how the environment contributes to more deliberate and focused thinking by Jane. There is an acknowledgement of the limitations of Jane's knowledge on a number of issues, but she is at last more in control of her thinking and, more importantly, of what she now intends to do. Priorities are being established, with some evidence of moving more purposefully towards some form of action. She still needs to remember her thoughts or, better still, to write a list of what she needs to do. At this point, after having made some personal decisions on which way to act, Jane will be limited until she finds the right moment to discuss things further with her colleagues.

The difference between routinely thinking and reflective thinking is that the former is relatively static and largely unresponsive to changing situations, while the latter involves a willingness to learn and change by purposefully going through the events, often some time after they have occurred. Conway (1994) helps to summarise this by describing reflection as: 'a process of looking back on what has been done and pondering on it and learning lessons from what did or did not work … the act of deliberation, when the practitioner consciously stops and thinks what shall I do now?'

Donald Schon (1991) describes two main types of reflection: reflecting-in-practice and reflection-on-practice. Reflecting-in-practice is where the practitioner has to think on his/her feet while the action is happening in practice. Reflection-on-practice is a more typical clinical supervision approach, where the supervisee looks back at a past event, e.g. caring for a particular patient/client, with a clinical supervisor. But reflection can also be used in clinical supervision as a rehearsal, e.g. reflecting with the clinical supervisor about how to interview somebody for the first time who has applied for a post on your ward. What has been described are three types of reflection, and all are apparent in Jane's situations (Box 2.1).

BOX 2.1	*Three different types of reflection based on Jane's activities*

- **While event(s) are happening**, e.g. while driving the car to work
- **After an event(s) has happened**, e.g. personal reactions and feelings about being questioned at the clinical supervision workshop
- **Before an event happens**, e.g. how to collect data from staff about their views on clinical supervision

Many of you reading this section of the chapter might now be thinking about something to do with clinical supervision in your practice area – what, exactly?

Keep the thoughts that have been stimulated by reading this part of the chapter in your head for a minute. How likely is it that they will they remain thoughts, or are you also working out ways you can put some of your thoughts into workable actions in practice? You are now beginning to use reflection … jot your thoughts down before you forget them!

HOW THE PROCESS OF REFLECTION RELATES TO THE PROCESS OF CLINICAL SUPERVISION

The process of reflection and the process of clinical supervision intersect at the point of wanting to intentionally learn something based on personal experience. In clinical supervision, it is the intention of the supervisee to learn something by sharing their experience of clinical practice with the clinical supervisor. Clinical supervision is therefore the mechanism by which safe, guided reflective practice can occur. As stated earlier, not all reflective practice is clinical supervision but potentially all good clinical supervision is reflective practice.

There are other mechanisms in clinical practice that offer an opportunity for reflection to occur (Box 2.2); you can probably think of other examples.

Many of the opportunities for reflecting about clinical practice are probably not too focused and the chances are that, while there may be an intention to

BOX 2.2	*Mechanisms in clinical practice where reflection can occur*

- Handover times
- Telephone conversations
- Teaching sessions
- Watching a video
- Reading a journal article
- Clinical case notes
- Case conferences
- Staff meetings
- Attendance at doctors' rounds
- The ward events or communications diary
- Working with nurses who are new to the healthcare setting
- Letters of complaint
- Critical or significant happenings on the ward/community settings
- Accident and near-misses forms
- The staff restaurant or rest room

learn, there is little follow-up on what actions arose from spending the time reflecting on practice. Talking, listening and reading can be helpful mediums for reflection, but are more powerful if shared with others rather than keeping things to yourself.

In your own personal experience and based on what you have read so far, how much reflection actually goes on at these times in clinical practice?

Regular clinical supervision offers continuity for the supervisee to focus on specific aspects of practice in an unhurried way. More importantly, it is also a mechanism for following up supervisee learning from sharing personal clinical experiences: in particular, what actions (if any) have been taken since the last clinical supervision session. The ability of the clinical supervisor to offer continuity for the supervisee's practice is lessened if what is spoken about during the session is forgotten by the next meeting.

Writing, whether it takes the form of reflective diaries or journals, is a powerful medium for facilitating reflection on practice (Walker 1985, Holly 1989, Kottkamp 1990, Patterson 1994, Street 1995, Fonteyn & Cahill 1998, Heath 1998) and assists the supervision process by acting as a reminder and a more in-depth analysis of what went on in practice (Fisher 1996). Apart from being a useful aide-memoire about clinical practice, recorded documentation of what goes on in the clinical supervision session is essential and, in a later chapter, is proposed as one of the responsibilities of the clinical supervisee. Reflective writing as a preparation for the session, or as a postsession activity, allows both the supervisee and supervisor to follow up on any intentions for practice and is a useful tool for monitoring the effectiveness of clinical supervision.

If the actions of reflection embody some change in the way somebody previously practised, there will also be consequences for the supervisee (Box 2.3).

BOX 2.3	*Possible consequences of being reflective in practice in clinical supervision*

- Standing out from the crowd
- Challenging conformity
- Often being a lone voice
- Not being satisfied with the way practice is carried out
- Wanting to find out more about why things are done in a particular way
- Being labelled a troublemaker
- Suggesting alternative ways of working
- Often being faced with making difficult choices
- Not having a knowledge of how to proceed with an idea
- Having more questions than answers
- Finding that others do not have answers to practice concerns
- Experiencing peer pressure to keep things as they are
- Afraid of rocking the boat in relation to future promotion or ambitions

Perhaps this is another reason why some practitioners find it difficult to reflect on their practice, preferring to just think about it in a superficial way. It may also explain why, in some introductory workshops, supervisees are initially reluctant to start the clinical supervision process. The role of the clinical supervisor in supporting and guiding any change the supervisee may be considering in their practice is therefore crucial, and is an important aspect of supervisor development and training. Perhaps there is also a mediation role for the clinical supervisor when critical incidents are replayed and difficult decisions have to be made.

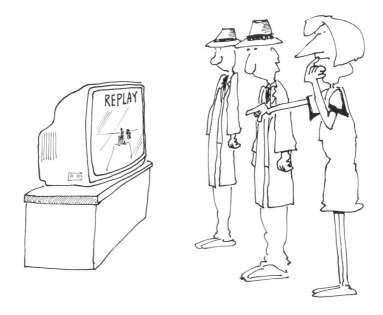

Chris Johns (1996) continues the theme of how challenging it can be, when formally reflecting on practice experiences, for practitioners to accept what is happening. His definition could have almost been written solely for the clinical supervision encounter:

> Reflection-on-experience is a window for practitioners to look inside and know who they are as they strive towards understanding and realising the meaning of desirable work in their everyday practices. The practitioner must expose, confront and understand the contradictions, within their practice, between what is practised and what is desirable. It is the conflict of contradiction and the commitment to achieve desirable work that empowers the practitioner to take action to appropriately resolve these contradictions (Johns 1996).

All practitioners/supervisees have some idea of what 'desirable practice' means to them individually and would, if they had the opportunity or the resources, want to work in that particular way. Personal conflicts often occur for practitioners when they become aware of the contradictions between how they would like to practise and how they actually do. Examining some of the contradictions that exist in practice, with someone else who understands that practice, coupled with a commitment to action, is the transformatory potential of clinical supervision described earlier. The commitment to action and attempt to reconstruct clinical practice is often the result of significant learning that has gone on in the clinical supervision session. 'My fears started to surface during my initial clinical supervision meetings. As I started to examine my interactions with my patients, it became clear that I consciously avoided forming any sort of relationship with the majority of them ... I was certain that I had the skills ... there just seemed to be a barrier which was preventing me from using them' (Moore & Carter 1998, p. 113).

Clinical supervision is concerned about reflecting not only on the big issues surrounding clinical practice but also on the seemingly insignificant and most ordinary of practice activities.

HOW BEING REFLECTIVE IN CLINICAL SUPERVISION CAN CHALLENGE ORDINARY PRACTICE ACTIVITIES

Anecdotally, I have noted how difficult it is sometimes for supervisees to recount ordinary stories from practice in clinical supervision. Instead, the content of a session is often something that made 'headline news', such as a patient complaint, something that went horribly wrong or a practice innovation. While these are all useful items to consider in clinical supervision, the supervisee can often become lost or seem insignificant in relation to them. When a supervisee is challenged to reflect on something ordinary, rather than extraordinary, that happened to them in practice, it is almost as if such things are not worth wasting supervision time on.

Read the account in the History Box of an activity I engage in every day – driving to work – to illustrate what I mean about 'ordinary' activities.

History Box

> I just couldn't be without my car. Living a good distance away from work results in a total travelling time of around 3 hours a day. Still, I'm not complaining I get a lot of satisfaction from doing what I do. I have to confess that driving has now become a routine activity during which I can also contemplate a session or meeting in the comfort of the car. In the car I often return to the supervision room and literally replay audio cassettes of what went on in my practice supervision. While listening to these hour-long cassettes, I also occasionally comment into a Dictaphone about what I consider significant aspects of supervision to write up later.
>
> It is while I have been in the supervision room (while driving) that I have been known to suddenly startle – you know that feeling when you wake up in the morning and realise the alarm has not gone off? I am suddenly thrust back into an awareness of being on the motorway, frantically looking for clues and landmarks that will reassure me that I have not missed the junction I wanted to leave at – perhaps having travelled for some time!

Reflective commentary

Not unlike Jane in the earlier example, the first part of my description of driving behaviour illustrates the number of different thoughts that go through my mind, instead of concentrating on what I am supposed to be doing, i.e. driving to work. My automatic thinking/action can be likened to what Tripp (1987) refers to as 'being on autopilot'. When I think back to how long it took me to learn how to drive a car – I failed my first test – nothing could be taken for granted in driving then.

It is interesting to note how many people I see on my travels engrossed in mobile telephone conversations, changing cassettes, hunting in a glove box for something while driving a car. I suppose, like me, when they first started to drive they had to concentrate on what they were doing if they wanted to pass the test and own a car. But what of them and me now? Is driving a car just a routine, or a potentially lethal activity? Perhaps with the emphasis on the safety specifications of cars as a major selling point, drivers now do not think too much about their own safety, believing that they will be able to survive any accident, what with side-impact reinforcing structures, rollcages and inflatable air bag devices.

Finally, and perhaps not surprisingly, more structured reflection was required on my part as I recently recounted the story of a minor accident to my insurance company over the telephone. This was followed by more formalised reflection on my driving behaviour, in the form of an insurance claim form and the use of drawings, before I could proceed with getting the damage repaired.

Although arduous, it forced me as a driver to think about my experience in a more structured way! In doing so, I became much more aware of my routine driving behaviour, as I actively described and analysed events surrounding the accident. I am now much more aware of my driving! If I can fail to acknowledge my routine driving behaviour, could the same complacency exist with what we might regard as 'routine' or everyday clinical practice(s)?

How many 'driving routines' like mine, occur in the delivery of your own clinical practice?
   What might be the consequences for you individually of not finding regular time to formally reflect on clinical practice in clinical supervision?

Interestingly, Professor Beverley Taylor (1994, p. 237) showed that, when nurses critically reflect on ordinary and everyday practice events in nursing, those same practitioners can become extraordinarily effective in contributing to patient outcomes. Johns (1995) concludes that the 'natural' tendency is for practitioners to pay attention to experiences that are disturbing to them in some way, leaving 'normal' practice not to be reflected upon because it is seemingly unproblematic. It is only by more actively noticing ourselves, e.g. my driving behaviour or your own behaviour in clinical practice, that we can become more able to actively learn and choose the next course of action. As one of the forefathers of reflective practice, John Dewey (1929, p. 367) succinctly stated: 'We do not learn by doing ... we learn by doing and realising what came of what we did'.

One would hope that realising what came of what we did does not occur in an intensive care unit as a result of a driving accident, or a disciplinary hearing as a result of a practice accident! By implication, being reflective also requires some form of action to follow the thinking and therefore presents supervisees, as well as the supervisor, with an opportunity to revisit existing practices and become a catalyst for change (Driscoll 1994, Ghaye et al 1996, p. 37).

Perhaps, as you consider the potential of taking regular time out to formally reflect on your practice in clinical supervision, you may prefer at first, as in a clinical supervision session, to have some form of structure to help you become more reflective in practice.

A MODEL OF STRUCTURED REFLECTION FOR THE CLINICAL SUPERVISION ENCOUNTER

When you look at the nursing literature, there are a number of reflective models to choose from (Benner 1984, Atkins & Murphy 1993, Shields 1994, Ghaye & Lillyman 1997, Johns 1997). More detailed reviews of reflection and reflective practice in nursing can be found in Atkins & Murphy (1993), Palmer et al (1994), Goff (1995a, 1995b), Clarke et al (1996) and Tsang 1998.

All reflective models are based on the premise that intentionally reflecting or learning about clinical practice will lead to a better understanding and awareness, thereby enhancing it.

That is what clinical supervision sets out to do. Clinical supervision is a form of guided reflection, in that it involves another person(s) helping someone to reflect about clinical practice during a session.

My revised What? model of structured reflection from an earlier publication (Driscoll 1994) contains three elements of reflection:

- **WHAT?** – a description of the event
- **SO WHAT?** – an analysis of the event
- **NOW WHAT?** – proposed actions following the event.

Each of the three elements interacts within the different stages of an experiential learning cycle (Figure 2.1).

| **Figure 2.1** | *The revised WHAT? model of structured reflection and its relationship to an experiential learning cycle* |

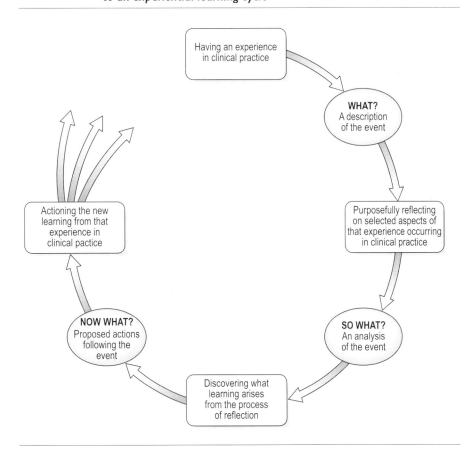

Associated trigger questions help in completing a learning cycle (Figure 2.2).

The What? model is not intended as a 'right way to reflect' but offers a structure for entering into a more meaningful exploration of events in clinical practice, either alone – e.g. while reading this book – or, preferably, with others in reflective supervision. The What? model of structured reflection can help a supervisee to prepare for clinical supervision and is discussed at length in Chapter 11.

While it is simplistic to suggest that considering a checklist of questions about clinical practice can transform it, the questions are intended to emphasise

| Figure 2.2 | The WHAT? model of structured reflection and associated trigger questions |

 A *description* of the event

WHAT? trigger questions:

- is the purpose of returning to this situation?
- happened?
- did I see/do?
- was my reaction to it?
- did other people do who were involved in this?

2 An *analysis* of the event

SO WHAT? trigger questions:

- How did I feel at the time of the event?
- Were those feelings I had any different from those of other people who were also involved at the time?
- Are my feelings now, after the event, any different from what I experienced at the time?
- Do I still feel troubled, if so, in what way?
- What were the effects of what I did (or did not do)?
- What positive aspects now emerge for me from the event that happened in practice?
- What have I noticed about my behaviour in practice by taking a more measured look at it?
- What observations does any person helping me to reflect on my practice make of the way I acted at the time?

3 Proposed *actions* following the event

NOW WHAT? trigger questions:

- What are the implications for me and others in clinical practice based on what I have described and analysed?
- What difference does it make if I choose to do nothing?
- Where can I get more information to face a similar situation again?
- How can I modify my practice if a similar situation was to happen again?
- What help do I need to help me 'action' the results of my reflections?
- Which aspect should be tackled first?
- How will I notice that I am any different in clinical practice?
- What is the main learning that I take from reflecting on my practice in this way?

practitioner learning and the subsequent actions that arise from them (if any). Many individuals may find that, after using the What? model of structured reflection, they wish to adapt or adopt more complex models of reflection as they become more familiar with the process. The original model came about as a response to learner nurses asking 'how do you reflect in practice?' (Driscoll 1994). With this newer version aimed at supervisees it can only ever be a guide. The emphasis in being a reflective practitioner, in whatever structure you find helpful to you, is on converting thinking about practice into some workable form of action. Stereotypically, you are likely to recount a negative aspect of your clinical practice in clinical supervision.

Find two sheets of A4 paper. Put as your main heading on one of the sheets the following phrase:

'Something that went well recently for me in practice was …'

or

'I really felt like a nurse in practice recently because …'

Using the What? model of structured reflection (Figure 2.2) to help you, describe (do not analyse), in as much detail as you can remember, the situation or event. You might just want to put in brief reminders, or phrases that were significant at the time, rather than write the whole story.

Next, take the other sheet of A4 paper and, again using the trigger questions to help you, analyse in more detail why you think such a good experience happened in your practice.

This exercise, if nothing else, is an example of the sort of learning activity you can include in a professional portfolio to maintain your registration. Most portfolios have space to write up reflective accounts. You may not have been altogether surprised to understand why the event went well. Chris Johns previously described reflection in terms of working towards desirable practice. An obvious conundrum to consider in conjunction with the above activity is why there are not more of these types of episode in clinical practice. How might they happen more often? Could this be real nursing knowledge for practice?

For the most part, clinical supervision is unlikely to consist of reflection on good aspects of practice with a clinical supervisor. Achieving desirable practice through reflection in clinical supervision is more likely to involve what hinders a practitioner from giving that desirable practice. The actions resulting from reflection will aim at what needs to happen to achieve quality care. Clinical supervision may well illustrate that it is not so often the organisation or the resources that are to blame. It may very well be the way in which practitioners organise and go about their nursing work.

IS REFLECTIVE PRACTICE THE ESSENCE OF CLINICAL SUPERVISION?

If you completed the previous activity you will realise that reflective practice is an intentional event and takes both time and commitment. What made you complete the activity? The answer to this question will form part of the conditions necessary for regular clinical supervision to occur. Alternatively, if you chose not to do the activity, what were your reasons? These may similarly form part of the obstacles to regular clinical supervision.

Transforming clinical practice through reflection is not yet an everyday activity. While it is liberating to learn from and alter the way we act in practice, unlearning what we have routinely been doing requires practical support as well as the courage to try. For the clinical supervision process to be effective it requires that the clinical supervisee/supervisor is interested in developing the necessary skills and attributes to be reflective in practice (Figure 2.3).

| Figure 2.3 | Reflective skills and attributes required for effective clinical supervision |

Clinical supervisor   Clinical supervisee

A willingness to learn from what happens in practice
Being open enough to share elements of practice with other people
Being motivated enough to replay aspects of clinical practice
Knowledge for clinical practice can emerge from within, as well as outside clinical practice
Being aware of the conditions necessary for reflection to occur
A belief that it is possible to change as a practitioner
The ability to describe in detail before analysing practice problems
Recognising the consequences of reflection
The ability to articulate what happens in practice
A belief that there is no end point in learning about practice
Not being defensive about what other people notice about one's practice
Being courageous enough to act on reflection
Working out schemes to personally action what has been learned
Being honest in describing clinical practice to others

Clinical
supervision

As Fish & Twinn rightly point out:

> any systematic approach to reflection can be used to investigate and theorise about practice ... but reflection does presuppose a seeking rather than a knowing attitude to practice and requires a practitioner to be open to criticism and to the possible need to change ... what it does not do, is to provide a clear set of detailed instructions for carrying out new practice (Fish & Twinn 1997, p. 69).

Instead it is likely that further reflection will be required to cope with the new challenges presented by 'relearning' clinical practice through clinical supervision. The 'qualified practitioner as learner' concept (Ghaye et al 1996, p. 6), requires supervisees to want to actively participate in their own learning and to consider ways of applying that learning back into practice. For supervisors, the process is about facilitating change in individuals by creating choices and options in practice, rather than telling the supervisee what to do from the basis of the supervisor's view of practice (Driscoll 1999).

A practitioner comment cited in one of the pioneering units developing and implementing clinical supervision in practice illustrates this:

> It's easy on a ward like this, or any other ward, to just sit back and whinge about things and I think what supervision certainly does for me is encourage me to actually tackle these things I'm whingeing about and to try and change things. It gives me that motivation and guidance (Kohner 1994, p. 24).

Wanting to realise desirable practice and believing that learning has no end-point is also just as important at the top as it is at the lower end of healthcare organisations. The actions of senior staff in supporting practitioners who wish to be more reflective in practice is more important than the production of nicely worded clinical supervision policy documents. The notion of a learning culture in clinical practice, one in which there is freedom to learn through reflection as well as do the work, must be a longer-term goal for an organisation if clinical supervision is to be fully implemented and is central to quality healthcare provision (Department of Health 1998).

Finally, it is my view that reflective practice is the essence of clinical supervision. Although it might be tempting to become a passive learner of someone else's ideas about clinical supervision, e.g. by reading a book like this, adopting a more reflective and critical approach to clinical supervision will make the initiative make more sense wherever you practice.

Do you think that reflective practice is the essence of clinical supervision? If so, what do you intend to now do about clinical supervision in where you work?

I would like now to invite you to reflect on what you have learned about reflective practice and clinical supervision in this chapter, which will become a template for helping you discover (and I hope learn) about clinical supervision throughout this book.

On reflection ... chapter summary

What are the key elements of this chapter?

- While not all reflective practice is clinical supervision, all clinical supervision is reflective practice
- It might be possible to transform nursing through the subsequent actions of being reflective in clinical supervision
- Clinical supervision is a legitimate opportunity for practitioners to stop and think about clinical practice
- Reflective learning differs from just thinking about clinical practice
- Writing about practice can assist the supervision process
- It can be useful to reflect on ordinary as well as extraordinary practice events in clinical supervision
- It can be helpful to consider some structure for engaging in critical reflection about practice
- Reflective practice requires time and commitment and is not an accidental event
- Monitoring the effectiveness of clinical supervision should be one of the first, not last, things to consider in any project

So what difference does this make to the way I am operating my clinical/ supervisory practice?

Now what actions will need to be taken as a result of my reflections?

REFERENCES

Atkins S, Murphy K 1993 Reflection: a review of the literature. Journal of Advanced Nursing 18: 1188–1192

Benner P 1984 From novice to expert: excellence and power in clinical nursing practice. Addison Wesley, Menlo Park, CA

Clarke B, James C, Kelly J 1996 Reflective practice: reviewing the issues and refocusing the debate. International Journal of Nursing Studies 33(2): 171–180

Conway J 1994 Reflection, the art and science of nursing and the theory–practice gap. British Journal of Nursing 3(1): 77–80

Dewey J 1929 Experience and nature. Grave Press, New York, p 367

Department of Health 1998 A First Class Service – Quality in the new NHS. Department of Health, London, UK

Driscoll JJ 1994 Reflective practice for practice – a framework of structured reflection for clinical areas. Senior Nurse 14(1): 47–50

Driscoll JJ 1999 Getting the most from clinical supervision: part two The supervisor. Mental Health Practice 3 (1): 31–37

Fish D, Twinn S 1997 Quality clinical supervision in the health care professions – principled approaches to practice. Butterworth-Heinemann, London

Fisher M 1996 Using reflective practice in clinical supervision. Professional Nurse 11(7): 443–444

Fonteyn ME, Cahill M 1998 The use of clinical logs to improve nursing students metacognition: a pilot study. Journal of Advanced Nursing 28 (1): 149–154

Ghaye T, Lillyman S 1997 Learning journals and critical incidents: reflective practice for health care professionals. Quay Books, Salisbury

Ghaye T, Cuthbert S, Danai K, Dennis D 1996 Learning through critical reflective practice. Book 5: Improving practice areas: practice in context. Pentaxion, Newcastle-upon-Tyne

Goff A 1995a Reflection – what is it? A literature review. Assignment 1(1): 7–14

Goff A 1995b Reflection – what is it? A literature review. Assignment 1(2): 24–28

Heath H 1998 Keeping a reflective practice diary: a practical guide. Nurse Education Today (18): 592–598

Holly ML 1989 Writing to grow: keeping a personal–professional journal. Heinemann, Portsmouth, NH

Jarvis P 1992 Reflective practice and nursing. Nurse Education Today (12): 174–181

Johns C 1995 The value of reflective practice for nursing. Journal of Clinical Nursing (4): 23–30

Johns C 1996 Visualising and realising caring in practice through guided reflection. Journal of Advanced Nursing (24): 1135–1143

Johns C 1997 Becoming an effective practitioner through guided reflection. PhD thesis, Open University

Johns C, Freshwater D (eds) 1998 Transforming nursing through reflective practice. Blackwell Science, Oxford

Kohner N 1994 Clinical supervision in practice. King's Fund Centre, London

Kottkamp R 1990 Means for facilitating reflection. Education and Urban Society 22(2): 182–203

Lumby J 1998 Transforming nursing through reflective practice. In: Johns C, Freshwater D (eds) Transforming nursing through reflective practice. Blackwell Science, Oxford, ch 8, p 91–103

Moore C, Carter J 1998 Exploration of the empowering potential of clinical supervision, reflection and action research. In: Johns C, Freshwater D (eds) Transforming nursing through reflective practice. Blackwell Science, Oxford, ch 9, p 104–118

Palmer A, Burns S, Bulman C 1994 Reflective practice in nursing – the growth of the reflective practitioner. Blackwell Scientific, Oxford

Patterson BL 1994 Developing and maintaining reflection in clinical journals. Nurse Education Today (4): 211–220

Reid B 1993 But we're doing it already! Exploring a response to the concept of reflective practice in order to improve its facilitation. Nurse Education Today 13(4): 305–309

Schon D 1991 The reflective practitioner – how professionals think in action. Avebury, Aldershot

Shields E 1994 A daily dose of reflection: developing reflective skills through journal writing. Professional Nurse 9(11): 755–758

Street A 1995 Nursing Replay – Researching Nursing Cultures Together (Ch 8 pp 147–171) Churchill Livingstone, Edinburgh

Taylor B 1994 Being human – ordinariness in nursing. Churchill Livingstone, Edinburgh

Tseng NM 1998 Re-examining reflection – a common issue of professional concern in social work, teacher and nursing education. Journal of Interprofessional Care 12 (1): 21–31

Tripp D 1987, cited in: Gray G, Pratt R (eds) 1994 Towards a discipline of nursing. Churchill Livingstone, Edinburgh, p 378

Walker D 1985 Writing and reflecting. In: Boud D, Keogh R, Walker D (eds) Reflection: turning experience into learning. Kogan Page, London, p 52–68

2 CLINICAL SUPERVISION IN PRACTICE

The purpose of Part 2 is to:

■ focus on clinical practice and ways in which clinical supervision can enhance the quality of that practice

■ consider how the practice of clinical supervision can contribute to the professional growth and development of the clinical supervisor as well as the supervisee

■ identify some of the skills and attributes required of the clinical supervisor and supervisee in practice and how both are dependent on the one another to maintain the initiative

■ empower those engaged in supervisory practice to consider and make choices as to what constitutes good clinical supervision

■ recognise what baseline elements of clinical practice might be considered therapeutic and how such skills could be noticed and translated into more effective clinical supervisory practice.

3 Is clinical supervision happening already?

INTRODUCTION

The previous chapter argued that learning is an intentional activity on the part of the practitioner but that formalising it outside the traditional classroom setting and within the culture of the clinical area is one of the biggest challenges facing clinical supervision. Although great things are expected of clinical supervision, it still has to compete with all the other things that make up the complex world of practice. This involves convincing sceptical practitioners that it is not simply a buzzword but that the time invested in it will be well spent.

This chapter sets the scene for the rest of the book as it moves away from the broader issues surrounding clinical supervision and becomes more practice-orientated. It begins with the premise that supervision is not a new thing in nursing, but that there are differences in its emphasis or function. The relationships that occur in supervision will therefore differ depending on what outcome is required.

Instead of adopting a new concept in nursing called clinical supervision, it might be useful to consider what is already happening in clinical practice that counts as supervision. In this way it will become evident that some of the skills already being used can be adapted to the supervision encounter.

TWO-DIMENSIONAL SUPERVISION

For many practitioners, clinical supervision begins in a formal classroom setting such as a training department or university college. In such an environment you often see 'traditional learners' arriving with big notepads and pens and seating themselves in the first available seat, often behind a desk. My own experience is that, when I invite the group to move the desks back and form a circle of chairs, there is some surprise that clinical supervision is not going to be taught 'at' them. The expectation of being 'taught' something new by someone who does not work in practice full-time has interesting parallels with clinical supervision. Further enquiry often reveals that many of the course participants have been sent 'kicking and screaming' on the course and that, not surprisingly, a number of preconceptions exist about what clinical supervision is about!

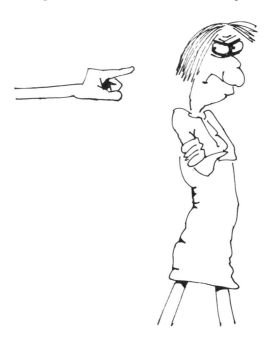

A general explanation of what clinical supervision is intended to be often elicits the by now familiar response to reflective practice: 'but we're doing that already!'

Nurses must be careful not to blindly adopt models of supervision as a convenient way of getting supervision in practice up and running (this theme is continued in later chapters). For instance, if we adopt the model of supervision used in the discipline of social work, three major differences come to mind straight away:

- Supervision is nearly always compulsory for social workers
- Social work supervision tends to be facilitated by immediate line managers
- Social workers are not self-regulating and do not yet have a statutory professional registration to maintain.

While the overall purpose of social work practice supervision might seem similar to the intention for nursing practice – e.g. safeguarding standards, supporting the practitioner and providing an opportunity to professionally develop – the context, and therefore the process of supervision, differs.

Seijo (1996, p. 41) develops the original work of Payne & Scott (1982) to describe social work supervision along two dimensions and can be a useful method of working out just where the place of supervision is likely to be in nursing practice (Figure 3.1).

Figure 3.1 *Two dimensional supervision (redrawn from Seijo H 1996 Developing supervision in teams: a workbook for supervisors. Association of Practitioners in Learning Disabilities, Nottingham, with kind permission of the publishers)*

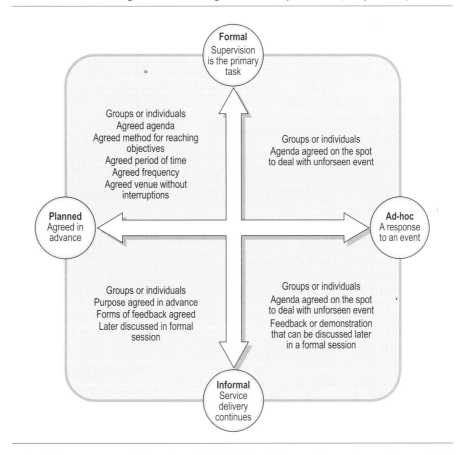

Looking at supervision through Seijo's different dimensions (Figure 3.1) gives an indication of the variable nature and roles of being a supervisor or being supervised. Supervisory activities are two-dimensional in that they can be 'formal' or 'informal' and 'planned' or 'ad-hoc'. The four quadrants that emerge illustrate the range and different types of supervisory activity going on in social work. They relate to the 'where' and 'when' of supervision. Particularly relevant for nursing practice is the upper right quadrant, which takes account of unexpected happenings that emerge outside planned supervision but could be a supervisory opportunity.

What activities already happen in clinical practice that might fit into each of the quadrants and perhaps count already as a form of supervision happening in nursing practice? Compare your ideas with Figure 3.2.

Figure 3.2   *Supervisory dimensions already happening in clinical nursing practice*

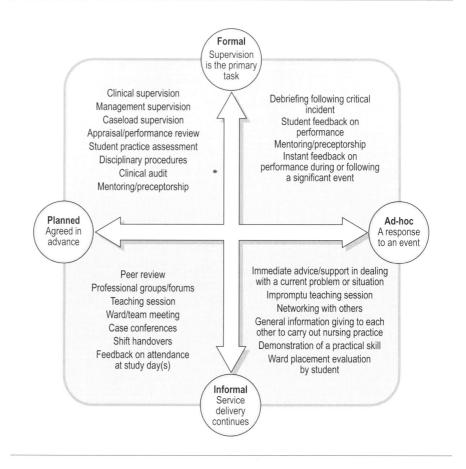

You may have been surprised to find that so many potential supervisory activities already happen in clinical practice, and at this stage this perhaps supports the notion that 'clinical supervision is already happening anyway'. I wonder how many readers agree that clinical supervision should be a formal and planned event, rather than being more flexible to accommodate the 'hurly-burly' of the clinical environment?

Perhaps it may be useful to initially make clinical supervision a prominent activity alongside those other activities, such as student assessment and regular meetings with the ward or unit manager, that it is impossible, or at least more difficult, to just quietly forget about. Clinical supervision should be regarded as an important and intentional activity, otherwise in practice when things get busy it will be the first thing to be dropped. How many good ideas can you think of that 'withered on the vine' because they only happened in an ad-hoc way or were seen as merely informal? In reality, the importance attached to clinical supervision will be decided not by those outside practice but by those inside practice who, after engaging in clinical supervision, value it enough to make it a prominent feature of clinical life.

THE COMPONENTS OF SUPERVISION IN NURSING PRACTICE

While clinical supervision may be a new concept to many practitioners, the three main components of it can be found in everyday practice:

- Supervised practice and learning
- Organisational supervision
- Supportive supervision.

Supervised clinical practice and learning

Fowler (1996) suggests, in his review of the literature, that the role of being a supervisor and assessor is well established within pre- and postregistration education. Both parties in this form of clinical supervision relationship operate in well-defined roles in which success takes the form of anticipated learning outcomes and a lot of ticked boxes and written comment. The supervisory role in this type of supervision is usually one of assessor and making sure that learners work in an area conducive to fulfilling the learning outcomes anticipated during their course of study.

Mentorship, despite the widespread use of the term in nursing, is often a confusing concept that lacks conformity nationally (Maggs 1994). Neary (1997), in a useful review, describes a mentoring role that can take the form of either a long- or a short-term relationship, in which the aim is to guide an assigned individual to a professional destination. She cites the key responsibilities as being responsible for the formalised teaching and assessment of learners but an adviser to staff already qualified (and presumably not on a course of study). Fowler (1996) perhaps summarises the vague nature of the mentor relationship best, as varying from a long-term nurturing and inspiring apprenticeship to being the person who shows you where to hang your coat and takes you to coffee.

What are some of the essential mentorship functions you already perform in practice? You can compare your ideas to those of Morton-Cooper & Palmer (1993, p. 63) in Box 3.1.

BOX 3.1	*The essential helper functions of mentoring (Morton-Cooper & Palmer 1993, p. 63)*

- **Adviser** – offering advice and support
- **Coach** – offering advice and instruction
- **Counsellor** – a listener and sounding board to encourage self-awareness
- **Guide/networker** – familiarisation with own contacts and power groups
- **Role model** – providing an observable image for imitation
- **Sponsor** – influencing others as to the mentee's potential at work
- **Teacher** – sharing knowledge through experience/facilitating learning
- **Resource facilitator** – providing access to available work resources

Aren't some of the things you are engaged in already, as a mentor in practice, transferable into the clinical supervision situation? Perhaps the roles or functions that you perform in clinical practice depend on what dimension of supervision you believe yourself to be in.

The introduction of PREPP (UKCC 1990) introduced the shorter-term relationship of the preceptor, providing a more orientating and supportive role to an individual nurse, midwife or health visitor who is, for whatever reason, new to the clinical environment, whether as a learner or as a newly qualified staff member. Fowler (1996) suggests that there is usually a teaching and assessment responsibility for learner nurses and a monitoring role for newly qualified staff.

Despite the obviously supportive nature of the preceptor role towards newly qualified staff (UKCC 1993), Philips et al (1996) argue that the terms 'mentor', 'preceptor' and 'supervisor' are often used interchangeably. This is not surprising, as even the supportive role of the preceptor involves assessing and recommending when the newly qualified nurse is ready to assume greater responsibilities. While it is beyond the scope of this text to debate and define the differing roles, substantial reviews can be found in Morton-Cooper & Palmer 1993, Maggs 1994, Jones 1996 and Butterworth 1998.

From your understanding and prior experience of participating in supervised practice as a mentor or preceptor:

■ What similarities and differences do you think there are between your existing role(s) and clinical supervision in practice, if introduced?

■ Can you think of any skills you already have that could be transferable into the clinical supervision situation?

Organisational supervision

As suggested in an earlier chapter, the term 'supervision', whether you are a charge nurse or a learner in practice, can conjure up images for the practitioner of being 'watched' or 'controlled' in some way by those responsible for the overall management of service delivery. Despite the great efforts that have been made to dissociate the professional development and supporting role of clinical supervision for already qualified clinical practitioners from more managerially led models of supervision, the substantive position paper on clinical supervision (Faugier & Butterworth 1994) was, as Bishop (1998, p. 1) notes, published on the very same day as the Clothier Report of the findings of the Allitt Inquiry (Department of Health 1994). This important document crystallised a number of concerns and made recommendations about the supervision of safe and accountable nursing practice.

Perhaps it is not altogether surprising that introductory clinical supervision workshops often have to manoeuvre through an initial stage of suspicion on the part of participants before they can examine the potential of regular clinical supervision in practice. There is no doubt of the need for a degree of managerial control in clinical practice (e.g. risk management, maintaining quality care, operationalising human resources, financial planning and associated activities) but managers should support not control the clinical supervision initative in practice. The legitimisation of regular time out to talk about clinical practice, I suspect, will be as much a challenge for practitioners who are used to being perpetually busy as it will be for managers to allow it to happen in work time.

The United Kingdom Central Council for Nursing, Midwifery and Health Visiting (UKCC 1996) unequivocally states that clinical supervision is not a managerial control system and is not:

- the exercise of overt managerial responsibility or managerial supervision
- a system of formal individual performance review
- hierarchical in nature.

Therefore the traditional aims and goals of management supervision, as a formal monitoring process that insists on good practice, differ from those of clinical supervision, which is a more enabling process supporting good practice. Undoubtedly, with resources scarce, clinical supervision may be influenced by those wishing for an efficient rather than necessarily an effective practitioner (Driscoll 1996). In other words, clinical supervision may be legitimised if it produces quantitative rather than qualitative outcomes. However as the UKCC (1996) again reminds those managers: 'By enabling practitioners to influence the development of clinical supervision, the resultant system can be trusted by all, avoiding the perception or actuality of management imposition'.

Supportive supervision

In order to survive the rigours of nursing practice, nurses have always created support systems. You may wish to compare again the different types of support detailed by Seijo (Figure 3.2) with your own practice. Some emerge almost intuitively, from working with and knowing that you can trust particular people, that they will not laugh at you and are prepared to listen to your concerns. Often, such encounters are ad-hoc and informal but play a vital part in coping with everyday clinical practice. Butterworth & Faugier (1992) describe these well-known ad-hoc and unplanned forms of supportive supervision as 'tear breaks' by means of which caring for one another can be an important way of surviving the business of caring for others.

The arguments Morton-Cooper & Palmer (1993, pp. 29–55) put forward for setting up more formal support structures in the clinical environment, such as preceptorship and mentoring schemes, also apply to the development of clinical supervision. The supportive roles of mentorship and preceptorship form the basis for clinical supervision partnerships:

- being accessible
- being responsive to other people
- being trusted
- being comfortable with one's own abilities
- having the respect of the other person(s).

Bishop (1994) is right when she states that, while a supportive, nurturing relationship for a novice practitioner (or someone new to the clinical area) is widely accepted in practice, it is not so readily accepted when the practitioner is no longer regarded as a novice. Perhaps you believe that such a relationship need not be necessary for an already accountable qualified nurse or health visitor in clinical practice?

THE SUPERVISION CONTINUUM IN NURSING PRACTICE

From the descriptions of the different types of supervision, a continuum of supervision emerges from within the organisational and career structures of nursing; this is summarised in Figure 3.3.

It begins with the supervised practice and learning of any unqualified or qualifying staff member, assessment of practice through mentorship schemes, a period of support, through preceptorship, on qualifying (or if new to the clinical environment), and formal as well as informal supported practice throughout one's clinical career.

Where would you place yourself on the supervision continuum? Do you agree that such supervision as is described here exists for you? Can you think of some examples that might illustrate what is meant by 'the supervision continuum' in nursing practice?

Fish & Twinn (1997, p. 16) make a useful distinction between two different modes of clinical supervision that for me validate the position of a supervision continuum in nursing practice and more clearly identify the differences and implications for clinical supervisory practice. The two modes they suggest have differing supervisory implications (Box 3.2).

The two modes described are a useful reminder of the concept of the lifelong learner, whether unqualified, qualifying or an experienced nurse professional. Mode 1 requires the supervisor to engage in some form of assessment of the learner, a term that includes both unqualified learners and qualified learners. Therefore, in this form of supervision there tends to be an unequal yet acceptable imbalance between the supervisor, who has the knowledge, experience and authority to be able to assess, and the learner, who is being assessed.

Mode 2 is significantly different, and is closely aligned with the ethos of clinical supervision that specifically relates to the professional development and support of an already qualified practitioner. Clinical supervision could be regarded not as the critical overseeing of another practitioner but as an intentional critical conversation to enhance practice, as defined by Wright: 'Supervision is a meeting between two or more people who have a declared interest in examining a piece of work. The work is presented and together they will think about what is happening and why, what has been done or said, and how it was handled – could it have been done better or differently and if so how?' (Wright 1989, p. 172).

Although supervision in practice often means meeting another person to talk about practice, Houston (1990) presents a number of different ways in which clinical supervision can be organised (Box 3.3).

| **Figure 3.3** | *Summary of the supervision continuum in nursing* |

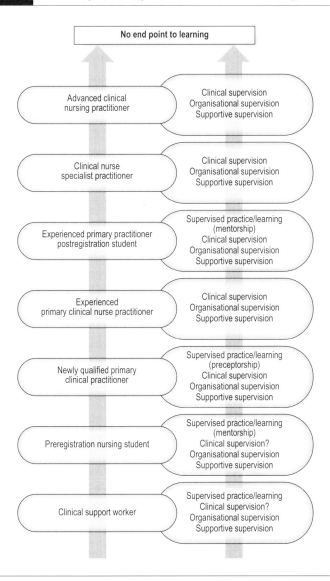

Probably in busy practice the key word is 'regular' and to achieve that will mean:

- clearing clinical supervision as a legitimate activity for work time with your line manager
- planning the time in advance
- looking around for possibilities that suit the way in which you work
- valuing the process of intentional critical conversations to enhance practice
- thinking of ways to demonstrate how clinical supervision sessions are effective or ineffective in the delivery of nursing
- viewing sessions as part of the normal learning activities of clinical staff.

| BOX 3.2 | *Supervisory implications of Fish & Twinn's (1997) two modes of clinical supervision* |

Mode 1: The on-course mode

The role of the clinical supervisor lies within the context of a professionally focused course and differs according to whether the supervision is:

- student supervision pre-Project-2000 (apprenticeship-type model)

or

- clinical supervision post-Project-2000 (towards a higher education degree- or diploma-type model, of which reflective practice has also been a feature).

Supervisory implications

- The needs of learners will differ significantly depending on the type of course they are undertaking
- Supervisors will need to reconsider, if traditionally trained, whether as supervisors they can fully meet the requirements of non-traditional methods of learning, e.g. facilitating reflective practice
- The supervisor may have responsibility for facilitating the learning and assessing the clinical competence of either preregistration learners or accountable and qualified practitioner learners
- The responsibility for formal assessment is a key aspect of the supervisory role in this mode

Mode 2: The professional development mode

Where supervisors work with qualified practitioners in the context of their daily work, they are clinically supervising already qualified practitioners who are not attending any formalised courses of academic study and their role differs according to whether the supervision is:

- the clinical supervision of staff who qualified prior to the implementation of Project 2000 (apprenticeship-type model)

or

- the clinical supervision of staff who qualified since Project 2000 (who already have a higher education degree or diploma or experience of reflective practice).

Supervisory implications

- The needs of the supervisee will differ depending on the type of course and learning experience undergone previously
- Supervisors may have to reconsider their methods of facilitating learning in others if they underwent an apprenticeship-type training to become nurses
- Depending on their experience, the supervisor has a different responsibility for facilitating the learning and continuing professional growth and development of qualified staff already accountable for their own clinical practice
- There is no formal assessment of a clinical colleague, who may be on an equal footing with the clinical supervisor in practice
- The previously agreed facilitation of reflective practice and giving feedback to colleagues on their clinical practice is a key aspect of the role of supervisor in this mode

BOX 3.3	*Different ways of organising clinical supervision in practice*

- Regular one-to-one sessions with a supervisor from the same discipline
- Regular one-to-one sessions with a supervisor from an allied discipline
- Regular one-to-one sessions with a peer/colleague supervisor
- Regular group supervision with a designated supervisor from the same discipline
- Regular group supervision with a designated supervisor from an allied discipline
- Regular group supervision with a designated peer/colleague supervisor
- Network supervision with those from a similar background or expertise who do not work together on a daily basis

At the end of the day it is important not to get too worried by how you organise the supervision at work but to try to ensure that some dedicated time is allocated to formally reflecting on practice with others. After all, it seems to happen already from an organisational and learning point of view, or when some form of support is needed, particularly when staff are not qualified or have not been qualified all that long. Why then is it not possible to extend this professional development and formal support to staff who have been qualified for some time? Could it be that such practitioners no longer need to learn about nursing?

IS CLINICAL SUPERVISION HAPPENING ALREADY – ADOPTION OR ADAPTATION?

There seem to be three main options for implementing clinical supervision in practice:

- Adopt other people's theories on clinical supervision, which reflect your way of working in clinical practice
- Adapt what you already have to fit in with accepted ideas of what clinical supervision is
- Do not even bother with such nonsense, because it happens already – doesn't it?

Whether clinical supervision is adopted or adapted, unless it is formalised and planned in its initial implementation it is unlikely to get off the ground. This is not to say that it cannot, if circumstances dictate, be carried out in the midst of everyday practice as well. The notion of 'live' (as it happens) supervision reduces the resources required and allows instant feedback on practice. But this method relies on one person (presumably the clinical supervisor) knowing more than the other (presumably the supervisee), and might turn out to be no more than just another form of supervised practice. The context and relationship of different forms of supervision also need consideration. Often this just means adjusting the hat you are wearing to suit the situation, by checking what your reason for supervising is and with whom you are engaging in it.

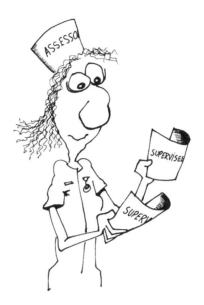

Look at Figure 3.4, which incorporates the supervision dimensions and continuum, as well as describing different structural aspects of clinical practice. See if it helps you to identify the different supervisory mechanisms that may already be operating in your place of work.

You may wish to consider the following questions alone, but it is preferable to involve others you work with:

- Where are you individually located on the supervision continuum?

- In what dimensions do you prefer to give supervision, and for what reasons?

- In what dimensions do you receive supervision (if at all), and for what reasons?

- In your opinion, is it appropriate for clinical supervision to be planned and formal?

- In what ways do you think clinical supervision differs from other forms of supervision that occur in your practice area?

- What sort of challenges may need to be overcome in practice to engage in clinical supervision as a clinical supervisor or supervisee?

- What evidence supports the notion that clinical supervision is happening already?

In response to the final question, I would suggest that locating clinical supervision within everyday clinical practice as a formalised and planned activity, particularly in adult nursing, would help to legitimise and protect the activity in an environment where there never seems to be enough time. Finding the time might be easier and clinical supervision might be more socially acceptable if it was seen as part of the everyday activities of the clinical area.

Figure 3.4 *Supervisory mechanisms in clinical nursing practice*

No end point to learning	Formal planned Supervision agreed in advance together	Informal ad-hoc Supervision as a reactive response to something	Informal planned Supervision planned after a happening	Formal ad-hoc Supervision within a working structure	Reflection on practice
Advanced clinical nursing practitioner (mode 1/2)	Clinical audit	Phoning a colleague for support with a situation they have previously experienced	Setting up a group to look into a recurring situation in the unit	Managerial feedback over lunch of availability of research monies	
Clinical nurse specialist practitioner (mode 1/2)	Caseload or management supervision	Networking with someone who visited the clinical area	Organising a case conference for unit staff	Discussion with visiting lecturer of student evaluations on teaching performance in college	
Experienced primary practitioner postregistration student (mode 1/2)	Mentorship from a colleague in practice for the duration of the course	General information seeking from a peer on the course working in the hospital	Discussing a new piece of research relevant to consider in the clinical area	Managerial feedback over coffee of the effects of ward project on the clinical staff	
Experienced primary clinical nurse practitioner (mode 1/2)	Annual appraisal and performance review	Asking a senior colleague to demonstrate a new technique	Discussion of a practice issue with a specialist practitioner over lunch	Debriefing with ward staff at handover of an unexpected death of a patient	
Newly qualified primary clinical practitioner (mode 2)	Agreed monthly preceptorship meeting	Seeking out advice or peer support in dealing with a new situation	Feeding back to colleagues at a monthly ward meeting the content of an attended study day	Feedback after a shift on how a situation was handled	
Preregistration nursing student (mode 2)	Practice, placement, assessment and evaluation	Impromptu teaching session	Verbally handing over allocated patients at the end of a shift	Feedback by clinical staff on performance during a busy shift	
Clinical support worker	Annual appraisal interview with charge nurse	Asking questions whilst observing a qualified nurse doing a task	Giving personal observations at a case conference	Giving of a professional opinion on how a situation was handled	
					The complexities of everyday clinical practice

The next chapter will explore the different frameworks that can be used during clinical supervision.

On reflection ... chapter summary

What are the key elements of this chapter?

- Different forms of supervision already exist in clinical nursing practice but need to be distinguished from clinical supervision

- Supervised clinical practice is not clinical supervision although some of the skills can be used by the clinical supervisor and supervisee

- Management supervision is different from clinical supervision

- Clinical supervision is aimed at helping qualified nurses enhance their clinical practice

- A supervision continuum already exists in nursing practice

- The on-course mode of clinical supervision has different supervisory implications from the professional development mode of clinical supervision

- The number of different ways of organising clinical supervision means it is adaptable into most forms of clinical practice

- It is debatable whether clinical supervision is happening already for qualified practitioners

So what difference does this make to the way I am carrying out my clinical/supervisory practice?

Now what actions will need to be taken as a result of my reflections?

REFERENCES

Bishop V 1994 Clinical supervision for an accountable profession. Nursing Times 90(39): 35–37

Bishop V (ed) 1998 Clinical supervision in practice – some questions, answers and guidelines. Macmillan/Nursing Times Research, London

Butterworth T 1998 Clinical supervision as an emerging idea in nursing. In: Butterworth T, Faugier J, Burnard P (eds) Clinical supervision and mentorship in nursing, 2nd edn. Stanley Thornes, Cheltenham

Butterworth T, Faugier J 1992 Clinical supervision and mentorship in nursing. Chapman & Hall, London

Department of Health 1994 The Allitt Inquiry. Independent inquiry relating to deaths and injuries on the Children's Ward at Grantham and Kesteven General Hospital during the period February to April 1991 (Clothier Report). HMSO, London

Driscoll JJ 1996 Reflection and the management of community nursing. British Journal of Community Health Nursing 1(2): 92–96

Faugier J, Butterworth T 1994 Clinical supervision: a position paper. School of Nursing Studies, University of Manchester, Manchester, p 1–60

Fish D, Twinn S 1997 Quality clinical supervision in the health care professions – principled approaches to practice. Butterworth-Heinemann, London

Fowler J 1996 The organisation of clinical supervision within the nursing profession: a review of the literature. Journal of Advanced Nursing (23): 471–478

Houston G 1990 Supervision and counselling. Rochester Foundation, London

Jones A 1996 Clinical supervision: a framework for practice. International Journal of Psychiatric Nursing Research 3(1): 290–308

Maggs C 1994 Mentorship in nursing and midwifery education: issues for research. Nurse Education Today (14): 22–29

Morton-Cooper A, Palmer A 1993 Introduction to support roles. In: Mentoring and preceptorship – a guide to support roles in clinical practice. Blackwell Science, Oxford

Neary M 1997 Defining the roles of assessors, mentors and supervisors. Part 1. Nursing Standard 11(42): 34–39

Payne C, Scott T 1982 Developing supervision of teams in field and residential social work. National Institute of Social Work, London

Philips RM, Davies WB, Neary M 1996 The practitioner teacher: a study in the introduction of mentors in the pre-registration nurse education programme in Wales. Part 2. Journal of Advanced Nursing (23): 1080–1088

Seijo H 1996 Developing supervision in teams: a workbook for supervisors. Association of Practitioners in Learning Disabilities, Nottingham

UKCC 1990 The report of the Post-Registration Education and Practice Project (PREPP). United Kingdom Central Council for Nursing, Midwifery and Health Visiting, London

UKCC 1993 The Council's position concerning a period of support and preceptorship for nurses, midwives and health visitors entering or re-entering registered practice (Annex 1 to Registrar's Letter 1/1993). United Kingdom Central Council for Nursing, Midwifery and Health Visiting, London

UKCC 1996 Position statement on clinical supervision for nursing and health visiting. United Kingdom Central Council for Nursing, Midwifery and Health Visiting, London

Wright H 1989 Groupwork: perspectives and practice. Scutari Press, London

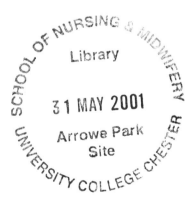

4 An interactive framework for supervisory practice

INTRODUCTION

In exploring the concept of clinical supervision, the previous chapter suggested that the components of clinical supervision might already be contained within the nursing work that is being done. The difficult part is eliciting, through critical reflection, not only what we do but how it happens in practice.

The complex nature of what and how we do things in clinical practice presents us with a contradiction in introducing clinical supervision in practice. Any framework used for clinical supervision in nursing needs to be comprehensive enough to straddle many different specialities but at the same time not so complex that practitioners cannot understand how to implement it in everyday practice.

Also as suggested in the last chapter, supervision in nursing can be viewed as constituting a continuum on which there is no endpoint to learning about clinical practice no matter how senior or experienced the practitioner. Taken like this, the introduction of clinical supervision could be viewed as 'topping up' existing skills and presenting learning opportunities for already qualified practitioners. This chapter's theme, and indeed the whole premise of the book, is that we can build on what we already have in practice rather than inventing something new and complicated.

Brigid Proctor's interactive model of supervision (Proctor 1986) features prominently in the nursing literature as a way of going about clinical supervision (Hughes & Morcom 1996, Bishop 1998, Butterworth et al 1998, Dolley et al 1998, Fowler 1998, Power 1999). Nicklin (1997) suggests that Proctor's work might already offer nurse practitioners a practice-centred model of clinical supervision, by virtue of what already happens in practice. Bowles & Young (1999) using Proctor as an evaluation tool in one NHS trust, are suggestive that nurses reported clear benefits in each of the components of Proctor's model in clinical supervision. Rafferty et al (1998)also used Proctor's framework to describe what was happening in clinical supervision, and even set standards in clinical supervision based on the model.

This chapter examines Proctor's interactive model of supervision starting from the premise that clinical practitioners already possess a range of different skills that are implicit within her framework. It also suggests that some of the skills practitioners may adapt for use in clinical supervision could be 'overused', restricting the dynamic nature of clinical supervision in practice.

THE PURPOSE OF CLINICAL SUPERVISION IN PRACTICE

In Chapter 1 I quoted Kohner's definition of clinical supervision as 'a formal arrangement enabling nurses to discuss their work regularly with another experienced professional … and involves reflecting on practice in order to learn from experience and improve competence' (Kohner 1994, p. 2).

This offers not only the 'how' of clinical supervision, but also the 'why'. Not surprisingly, it reflects the main aims of clinical supervision defined by Bishop (1994), as not only to benefit the person being 'supervised' but in doing so to offer a mechanism for improving the quality of patient care by:

- maintaining and safeguarding standards of care
- valuing the development of professional and practice knowledge
- ensuring the optimal delivery of quality care.

Therefore, any model of clinical supervision in nursing practice needs to take account of these primary aims. They are a useful starting point for laying out a testing ground for clinical supervision within clinical practice. Bearing these aims in mind, practitioners engaging in clinical supervision for the first time must also consider what likely benefits or outcomes there could be for:

- the individual nurse practitioner
- the recipient of nursing interventions by the nurse practitioner
- the institution within which nursing is practised.

In this way, the focus of clinical supervision sessions is always practice concerns, as the issues explored in supervision will always be from within the domain of clinical nursing. Regardless of any model of clinical supervision adopted, any positive outcomes or benefits will come directly from the practitioners themselves, who continually guide and shape the process.

Proctor's interactive model of supervision, then, must always be a tentative guide, which will no doubt over time be shaped or discarded by practitioners as they become more used to engaging in clinical supervision. One of the main advantages for practitioners of this framework, as suggested earlier, is that the component parts or functions of Proctor's model already exist in everyday nursing practice.

THE FUNCTIONS OF PROCTOR'S INTERACTIVE MODEL OF SUPERVISION

Proctor's interactive model of supervision (Proctor 1986) has three interactive functions (Figure 4.1), which relate to the role and function of the clinical supervisor but can also be used by the supervisee as a preparation for attending a clinical supervision session.

Figure 4.1   *The three functions of Proctor's interactive model of supervision*

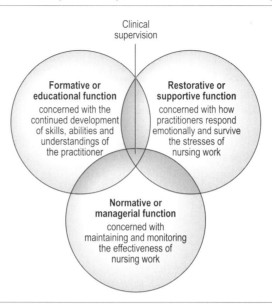

The three functions also give a focus to a clinical supervision session between the supervisor and supervisee (Box 4.1) and are not dissimilar to the supervisory functions discussed in the previous chapter – e.g. supervised practice, supportive supervision, organisational supervision.

BOX 4.1   *How Proctor's interactive model of supervision relates to the continuum of nursing practice (Chapter 3)*

A **formative** or **educational** function (supervised practice)
A more adult learning approach is adopted in clinical supervision whereby the clinical supervisor attempts to facilitate the supervisee's learning through supported and often guided (offering a structure) reflective practice. Ideally, preceptorship is the forerunner of clinical supervision.

A **restorative** or **supportive** function (supportive supervision)
While it certainly has been a long time in coming, support for practitioners while at work is a key feature of clinical supervision. To be effective, it requires that the supervisee trusts the clinical supervisor enough to disclose elements of clinical practice that are challenging and difficult in a caring, confidential and supportive environment. It is a planned rather than a reactive event in practice.

A **normative** or **managerial** function (organisational supervision)
While this is the most controversial function in relation to qualified practitioners, there are areas in nursing of high litigation risk in which a more directive approach is required or even mandatory, e.g. issues of child protection, sexual abuse or caseloads gauged alongside risk management criteria, as in mental health. In many cases this will involve giving advice or information to inexperienced practitioners rather than telling somebody what to do. This is distinct from managerial supervisory activities such as appraisal or formally disciplining an individual practitioner.

Proctor's clinical supervision model could be seen as a toolbox that you can dip into to build, prop up or reconstruct clinical practice

What **formative** or **educational** tools might you already have in your practice toolbox to do the job of nursing?

What **restorative** or **supportive** tools might you already have in your practice toolbox to do the job of nursing?

What **normative** or **managerial** tools might you already have in your practice toolbox to do the job of nursing?

Now compare your own thoughts with those of Richard a staff nurse who has been working in orthopaedics for just over a year and is currently using a number of supervisory tools (Box 4.2). While Richard would appear already to have a number of skills and attributes relating to the functions of clinical supervision, how useful might clinical supervision be for his practice?

BOX 4.2	*Different tools used by Richard for doing the job of nursing*

Formative or **educational** tools in use:

■ Able to teach and assess preregistration students in practice

■ Attendance at a recent study day on clinical supervision

■ Personal subscription to a relevant nursing journal

■ Starting to compile a personal profile and professional portfolio issued by the organisation to maintain professional registration

■ Membership of a monthly mentors and preceptors forum

■ Membership of a group reviewing nursing documentation

■ Certificated attendance at a manual handling update

■ Working with colleagues to devise an information leaflet on healthy eating for discharged patients following orthopaedic surgery

Restorative or **supportive** tools in use:

■ Recognises when he is beginning to feel pressured at work

■ Starting to be more open with a trusted staff colleague about the way he is feeling during a shift

■ Mainly relies on friends and family to offload difficult situations experienced in clinical practice

■ Feels more able to discuss at handover aspects of care he is not happy about and suggest ways forward

■ Responsible for collecting staff monies for the monthly ward meal at the local pizza house

■ Cited in evaluations as being a source of support to newly arrived students on the ward

■ Trusted by the ward manager to keep an eye on junior staff members who find the work initially difficult

| BOX 4.2 cont. | *Different tools used by Richard for doing the job of nursing* |

Normative or **managerial** tools in use:

- Participated in a recent audit measuring patient satisfaction with the clinical area
- Completed most of the objectives set last year at the induction interview
- Able to manage and prioritise clinical care for a group of patients, as well as on occasions to run the ward in the absence of the charge nurse
- More knowledgeable about organisational policies relating to patient and personnel safety on the ward
- Has experience of handling complaints with tact in the clinical area
- Has had personal experience of being complained about by a patient's relative (although unjustifiably) and interviewed formally by the ward manager
- Not frightened to offer a professional opinion to senior medical staff visiting the ward
- Aware of professional duties and responsibilities in relation to the UKCC code of professional conduct (UKCC 1992)

Imagine that you are a colleague on Richard's ward and that last week Richard approached you about being his clinical supervisor. You already know quite a bit about him already:

Case history

Richard qualified as a staff nurse just over a year ago. Although working on an orthopaedic ward now, Richard intends to specialise in Accident & Emergency when there is a vacancy in the department. While on the preregistration course he found that taking time out to reflect was time-consuming but a worthwhile activity. Nowadays his colleagues always seem to be too busy doing things to spend any time out talking with him about orthopaedic practice.

Richard is a bit disillusioned that he was not accepted directly into the Accident & Emergency Department after qualifying. Instead, he was advised to get some general ward experience first. Richard's line manager, Jean, has noticed that he seems to find time on the ward for student nurses' concerns but is often irritated by and spends little time with his peers. He remains a popular nurse with patients and is often sought out by worried relatives at visiting time.

Although he will not admit it, Richard still worries about how he will cope with a cardiac arrest situation involving a young adult on the ward. He has had some experience of dealing with cardiac arrests in elderly patients. On the one hand, cardiac arrests in young people are a rarity (thank goodness) but on the other hand, when they do happen Richard seems to be either on nights or having a day off. Richard feels that he would like to deal with a cardiac arrest in a young adult and see how he copes before reapplying for an Accident & Emergency post.

If you were his clinical supervisor, in what ways would Proctor's interactive model of supervision help you identify some of the blind spots in Richard's clinical practice?

There are a number of contradictory ideas involved in the last activity and clinical supervision. Had you begun to realise them? These will be explored in more detail in the next chapter.

The ideas that you came up with in the last exercise are yours as an imaginary supervisor and not necessarily what Richard might notice, see as significant or even wish to share with you, despite the fact that you are a colleague.

Some of the material is a bit sensitive and embarrassing for Richard.

What would your reaction be if you found out that Richard wanted to leave, assuming that you do not already know?

TRIANGLES IN CLINICAL SUPERVISION

Proctor's model of supervision may be compared with different models of nursing. In reality, the component parts merely represent the nurse theorist's preference or focus for delivering patient care – psychosocial, physiological, rehabilitative, etc. Using this model in the clinical supervision encounter may well be similar.

Although the three elements of supervision seem to apply equally, in reality, just as in different nursing theories, there will inevitably be unequal and overlapping functions in the supervision encounter. Hughes & Pengelly (1997) simplify the functions of clinical supervision, or what the clinical supervisor is trying to do, in the form of an equal triangle (Figure 4.2).

Figure 4.2	*A supervisory triangle based on what the supervisor attempts to do*

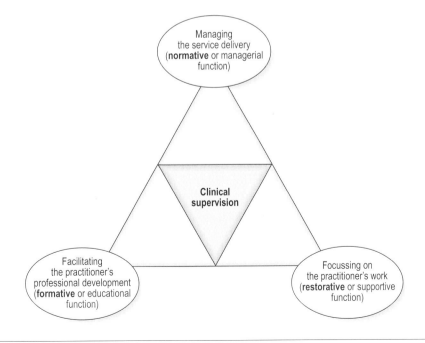

Going back to 'your own favoured way of seeing' somebody else's (Richard's) clinical practice, how did the 'equal' triangle of clinical supervision become distorted as you applied your own focus to Richard's situation as a potential clinical supervisor? Imagine the different combinations that potentially exist between you as a clinical supervisor and the supervisee coming for clinical supervision! As one point of the triangle is recognised and explored by the supervisor, so another point of the triangle can get left out or ignored completely (Figure 4.3).

| **Figure 4.3** | *A 'distorted' supervision triangle based on the clinical supervisor's favoured way of seeing the supervisee* |

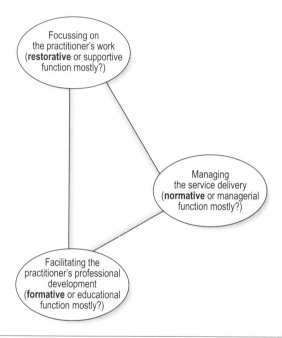

Often the area that is ignored in supervision is the component that the supervisor does not feel confident or skilled in. Instead of focusing on one's own area of expertise (look at your own comments from the previous thinking exercise), the clinical supervisor and supervisee can both learn from trying to give equal time and space to each of Proctor's primary functions of clinical supervision:

- normative (managerial/organisational function)
- formative (learning/educational function)
- restorative (supportive function).

This raises interesting questions about the different types of supervision that already exist in nursing practice not just between qualified and unqualified staff, but between different postqualification levels of expertise and experience. I think that it also validates some of the points raised in the last chapter about the suggestion that a continuum of supervision in nursing already exists in practice.

PULLING IT ALL TOGETHER: POSSIBILITIES FOR CLINICAL SUPERVISION SESSIONS

Clinical supervision is a complex activity that can allow routine everyday clinical practice to be seen through different lenses. Although Proctor's interactive model of supervision is useful for breaking down supervision into its component parts, it does not cover all situations faced in clinical supervision.

It is useful from a structural point of view to remind practitioners of the broader aspects of clinical practice that are not often thought about very much because of the pressures of delivering a health service on a daily basis. It may be possible to evaluate to what extent the different functions of clinical supervision are addressed in sessions and compare this with the overall delivery of service and see what, if any, aspects of clinical practice are enhanced, either for a whole group of clinicians or for an individual.

Being aware of the different functions and possibilities of supervision is not only useful to the clinical supervisor for structuring or producing criteria for supervision, but also to the supervisee for maximising the use of the session time available. Clinical managers will also need convincing that clinical supervision is more than a cup of tea and a cigarette while practitioners get out of doing the work and leave colleagues to struggle. Articulating the functions of clinical supervision using Proctor's framework is a useful baseline from which to start.

For instance, Bowles & Young (1999) developed a clinical supervision measurement tool, based on Proctor, that will contribute to the emerging taxonomy of clinical supervision outcomes in practice. Rafferty and his colleagues (1998) adapted Proctor's model to form the basis of a telephone survey in mid- and west Wales that aimed to find out just what was happening on the clinical supervision front, and even began setting standards for clinical supervision using the framework (Chapter 11). Instead of using the concepts of Formative–Normative–Restorative, they simplified them as Learning–Accountability–Supportive to make them easier to understand.

Keep a small journal to note down when individual staff (or even yourself) use one another:

- restoratively
- normatively
- formatively.

You can access this information using the trigger questions in Box 4.3 either to check what is happening in your own clinical supervision sessions or alternatively to detect elements of clinical supervision already happening in your clinical area.

It may also be possible to consider the different functions of supervision and how much one of the functions is avoided or overused by yourself or others in clinical practice. Do any of these functions tend to be used by staff with patients/clients?

| BOX 4.3 | *Detecting elements of clinical supervision in everyday practice* |

- What do others say or do that makes you think they are using one of Proctor's supervisory components?
- Who initiates it and how is it done?
- Does the person who initiates the activity usually get the desired outcome?
- How much of this is dependent on the other person?
- Is it possible to block the function being performed?
- How is this done?
- Do certain members of staff, in your opinion, overuse any of the functions, for example always being normative and directive?
- Do certain members of staff, in your opinion, seem to actively avoid any of the functions, for example never to use supportive functions?
- How do you feel yourself when people use this function on you?
- What do you like or dislike about the way the function is performed on you in everyday clinical practice?
- What can you learn from these observations to use in your own supervision, whether as a supervisor or supervisee?
- How do patients/clients tend to react to staff using such functions?

In clinical supervision workshops I often use a 30-minute role-play as a snapshot of a clinical supervision session. Each of the observers has to give feedback to the main players based on different aspects of supervisory practice. Often, observers take one component of Proctor's model and observe the different types of interaction/intervention in supervisory practice. While it is not ethically sound to sit in on somebody else's supervision session to observe the different functions, they can be seen in everyday clinical practice, although not as clinical supervision.

The next chapter discusses how important it is to be specific about the roles and responsibilities the supervisor and supervisee have towards each other in the supervisory partnership. This chapter reminds practitioners that, when clinical supervision starts off, either the supervisee or the supervisor may adopt their 'normal' or 'usual' roles in clinical practice. But, as we have seen, this may be entirely inappropriate in the clinical supervision session, suggesting that Proctor's interactive model of supervision may be of use in preparing for the new roles of clinical supervisor or supervisee. It is also important that roles and responsibilities include an element of negotiation about what is expected of each of you, in the form of a contract. This is usually the basis for getting started in the first session, after you have sat looking at each other a bit awkwardly for the first few moments!

On reflection ... chapter summary

What are the key elements of this chapter?

- To be useful for practice, clinical supervision has to be grounded in practice

- Clinical supervision is a purposeful activity that, if functioning properly, not only benefits staff but also enhances clinical practice

- Any model of clinical supervision in practice can only be tentative at present

- Proctor's interactive model of supervision appears to have been widely adopted where supervision is used in clinical practice

- Proctor's interactive model of supervision identifies functions of supervision that provide a framework for the supervisee to use as well as the supervisor

- Both supervisors and supervisees may prefer some functions to others

- Proctor's interactive model of supervision is unlikely to cover every aspect of supervisory practice

- Some of the components of Proctor's interactive model of supervision can be observed in practice already

So what difference does this make to the way I am operating my clinical/supervisory practice?

Now what actions will need to be taken as a result of my reflections?

REFERENCES

Bishop V 1994 Clinical supervision for an accountable profession. Nursing Times 90(39): 35–37

Bishop V (ed) 1998 Clinical supervision in practice – some questions, answers and guidelines. Macmillan/Nursing Times Research, London

Bowles N, Young C 1999 An evaluative study of clinical supervision based on Proctor's three function interactive model. Journal of Advanced Nursing 30(4): 958–964

Butterworth T, Faugier J, Burnard P (eds) 1998 Clinical supervision and mentorship in nursing, 2nd edn. Stanley Thornes, Cheltenham

Dolley J, Davies C, Murray P 1998 Clinical supervision: a development pack for nurses (K509). Open University Press, Buckingham

Fowler J (ed) 1998 The handbook of clinical supervision – your questions answered. Quay Books, Salisbury

Hughes R, Morcom C 1996 Clinical supervision – distance learning package. Warrington Community Health Care (NHS) Trust, Warrington

Hughes L, Pengelly P 1997 Staff supervision in a turbulent environment – managing process and task in front-line services. Jessica Kingsley, London

Kohner N 1994 Clinical supervision in practice. King's Fund Centre, London

Nicklin P 1997 A practice centred model of clinical supervision. Nursing Times 93(46): 52–54

Power S 1999 Nursing Supervision: a guide for clinical practice Ch 2 pp 17–32, Sage, London, UK

Proctor B 1986 Supervision: a co-operative exercise in accountability. In: Marken M, Payne M (eds) Enabling and ensuring – supervision in practice. National Youth Bureau, Council for Education and Training in Youth and Community Work, Leicester, p 21–34

Rafferty M, Jenkins E, Parke S 1998 Clinical supervision: what's happening in practice? A report submitted to the Clinical Effectiveness Support Unit (Wales). School of Health Science, University of Wales, Swansea

UKCC 1992 Code of professional conduct. United Kingdom Central Council for Nursing, Midwifery and Health Visiting, London

5 Roles and responsibilities in clinical supervision

INTRODUCTION

This chapter reviews the shared and differing roles of the supervisee and supervisor in clinical supervision and their responsibilities to each other. In addition, for clinical supervision to be sustained in practice, front line managers also have roles and responsibilities to enable supervision to take place and provide an infrastructure for it.

It is suggested that a precontractual meeting is held to informally discuss what clinical supervision is, as well as what it is not, as a way for the parties to get to know one another before a supervision contract is drawn up. Although clinical supervision may take place in groups, the emphasis of this chapter will, however, be on the one-to-one encounter.

The first session will be analysed in detail, including some of the main points to consider in drawing up a supervision agreement or contract. It is argued that, for clinical supervision to be effective, the contractual elements agreed in the first session will form the basis of the supervisory relationship. If the parameters of clinical supervision are clearly set out, both the supervisor and supervisee can then begin to look at the supervisory opportunities and different ways of organising future sessions together.

CONTRACTING IN CLINICAL SUPERVISION

A supervision contract is arguably one of the most essential ingredients for the success of the supervisory relationship. The contract is a negotiated agreement that identifies ground rules about the supervision process (Gadd & Mahood 1995, p. 13). The United Kingdom Central Council for Nursing, Midwifery and Health Visiting (UKCC 1996) endorses the use of contracting in clinical supervision to establish what clinical supervision is and what it is not:

Ground rules need to be comprehensive and written down so that practitioners and supervisors are fully aware of the purpose and benefits of supervision. This includes stating how issues are raised, discussed or recorded and how confidentiality is dealt with. Written records of supervisory sessions are confidential and should only be disclosed with the consent of the supervisee. If clinical supervision is included in employment contracts, records may be requested by employers.

However, the fact that conditions might exist for clinical supervision in professional nursing does not necessarily mean that this will be shared by those engaging in it. For engagement to occur in clinical supervision between the supervisor and supervisee Morrison (1996, p. 31) suggests that there must be:

'a shared perception of, and commitment towards, supervision by both parties, based on clarity about agreed roles, responsibilities and expectations, and some understanding of the relevant past that each brings to the supervisory process'.

Morrison then insightfully states: 'If we don't understand where we are each coming from, we won't start together and may never catch up with one another!'

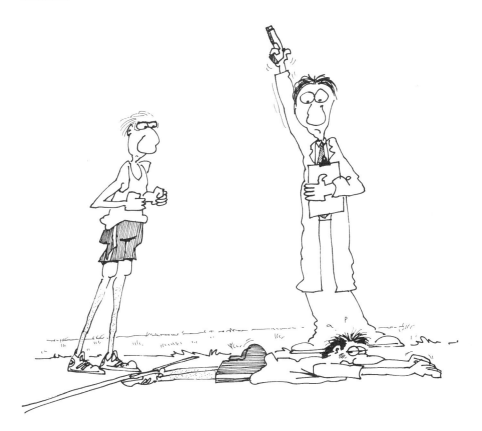

A precontractual meeting between the supervisor and supervisee can be helpful to explore each other's hopes, fears and expectations about clinical supervision. In many instances you may, as a supervisee, already know or even be able to choose your clinical supervisor and perhaps find the process a bit less daunting. Even so, it can be an interesting experience to consider the 'supervisory baggage' you will both be bringing with you into the clinical supervision room *before* you formally agree to engage in clinical supervision. Finding out how the other person's view of clinical supervision differs from yours begins the process of mutual trust by uncovering possible limitations to supervision and areas of learning for both of you.

What sorts of 'supervisory baggage' to do with clinical supervision might you be carrying that might need to be left outside the clinical supervision room?
Compare your ideas to those in Box 5.1.

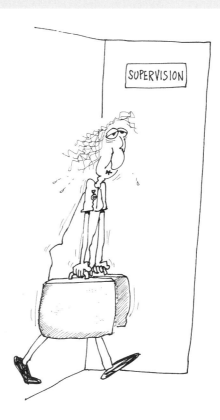

BOX 5.1	*Supervisory 'baggage' that might need to be left outside the clinical supervision room*

Previous experiences from being on the supervisory continuum in nursing, e.g. preceptorship, mentorship, being assessed in practice, appraisal interviews, etc. Often such experiences may be negative, the focus tending to be on what a person did wrong:

- 'The other person kept me hanging around for ages before they appeared'
- 'They never seemed to listen'
- 'There was never enough time to do anything constructive'
- 'We were always being interrupted'
- 'I didn't like the way I was spoken to'
- 'The person always managed to get my back up'

Agreeing a contract in clinical supervision is an essential part of sharing the ownership of it. Following such discussions, which are often the focus of the first session in clinical supervision, the contract clearly indicates what is intended to happen but, more importantly, it is suggestive of roles and responsibilities that will emerge after the agreement is signed. After all, signing a credit agreement for a new venture such as a new television or hi-fi system means that both parties can seek some redress if either is unhappy with a situation – but only with reference to what has previously been agreed. If there is no previous agreement, or boundaries, then anything could happen, and not necessarily for the best!

Brown & Bourne (1996, p. 50) rightly warn that getting the contract right does not guarantee successful supervision, but it does provide a firm foundation for more effective work. One of the ways it does this is by clarifying the specific roles and responsibilities each party will have in relation to clinical supervision, thus giving the opportunity at least to change what is going on. There are disadvantages in simply adopting a written contract produced by an organisation ('here's one we prepared earlier'), as this can reduce the sense of engaging in something that was agreed together. Most organisations suggest broadly headed contracts that are completed and signed at the end of the first session (Figures 5.1A–C).

Interestingly, one of the examples (Figure 5.1C) tries to get the supervisee and supervisor to think of the contract in terms of individual roles and responsibilities, as well as identifying shared responsibilities that will form the basis of clinical supervision. Fuller reviews of contracting in supervision can be found in Brown & Bourne (1996), Morrison (1996), Bond & Holland (1998), Dolley et al (1998), West Midlands Clinical Supervision Learning Set (1998) and Power (1999).

CONTRACTUAL ELEMENTS TO CONSIDER IN CLINICAL SUPERVISION

Box 5.2 identifies key issues to consider when contracting in clinical supervision. The contract must take into account **the purpose of clinical supervision and knowing what it is not**. It will be the exception, rather than the rule, particularly in adult nursing, if either the supervisor or supervisee has much experience in clinical supervision. More probably they will have previous experiences of supervised practice, preceptorship, mentorship, management or research supervision, which may be part of the 'supervisory baggage' alluded to earlier. Some erroneous models of supervision may well arise when contracting in clinical supervision for the first time. These models adapted from Bailey 1997 are listed in Box 5.3 and are indicators of a lack of understanding from either party, but particularly an inadequately prepared supervisor.

BOX 5.2	*Contractual issues to consider in clinical supervision*
	■ The purpose of clinical supervision and knowing what it is not
	■ Obtaining agreement on how sessions will be organised
	■ How participants will know if clinical supervision is working or not

Figure 5.1A   *An example of a clinical supervision contract*

⊛ BHB
COMMUNITY HEALTH CARE

Supervision contract   1998

Supervisee: ....

Supervisor: ....

Date contract agreed   ....
Date of review   ....
Frequency of supervision   ....
Duration of supervision   ....
Location   ....

Formations - individual, pair or team supervision:

Objectives of supervision - to discuss items relating to the following areas:

Confidentiality: -

Record keeping: -

Expectations: -

• an alternative date will be arranged by the party who cancels.
• each party will prepare their own agenda before the session.
• sessions will not be interrupted unless agreed beforehand.
• discussions will be open and honest.
• supervisee will provide information relating to work activities as appropriate.

Other issues

Signatures .... (Supervisor)
           .... (Supervisee)

The following two examples illustrate contrasting ways of introducing the contract between the supervisor and supervisee.

Supervisor: Thank you for coming to see me this afternoon, I think we had better start by getting this contract out of the way before I can begin supervision....

Supervisee: OK – where do you want to start?

Figure 5.1B	*An example of a clinical supervision contract*

Faculty of Health

CLINICAL SUPERVISION CONTRACT

Supervisee:
Supervisor:

Review date for evaluation of supervison:

Frequency/Duration of meetings:

Venue:

Maintaining confidentiality/Method of recording supervision sessions:

Guidelines for cancellation of planned supervision session:

Issues considered not appropriate for supervision:

WHAT THE SUPERVISEE EXPECTS FROM CLINICAL SUPERVISION:

WHAT THE SUPERVISOR EXPECTS FROM CLINICAL SUPERVISION:

Signature of clinical supervisor ....

Signature of clinical supervisee ....

Date: ....

Alternatively:

Supervisor: I'm glad we could both meet for our first clinical supervision together.... Don't worry, I'm probably more nervous than you. As I explained to you, I only did the course 4 weeks ago so we are both in a position of learning. It would probably be useful if we started by looking at what we expect from one another in supervision....

Supervisee: Well I've never been in supervision before, but in the supervisee workshop it was my understanding that this was my time to look at issues that are important to me.... I hope to use the time to ...

Figure 5.1C   *An example of a clinical supervision contract*

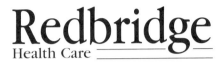

Redbridge
Health Care

Clinical Supervision Contract

Name/Designation (Supervisee): ....Date.................
Name/Designation (Supervisor): ....Date.................

The Clinical Supervisee and Supervisor take shared responsibility for:

As Supervisor, I take responsibility for:

As Supervisee, I take responsibility for:

The resource implications of supervision, particularly those of time and freeing up staff from clinical practice, will mean that managers, not unreasonably, will expect clinical supervision to be more than time out for a cup of tea. Professional expectations are that engaging in clinical supervision will enhance the work of practitioners and safeguard standards of patient care. Without some form of evidence to support this, it is very unlikely that clinical supervision will be allowed to continue.

Strategic organisational roles and responsibilities are aimed at providing training and an infrastructure to help practitioners get started in practice. Interaction between practitioners also involves roles and responsibilities. Box 5.4 illustrates the individual and shared roles and responsibilities of the supervisee and supervisor in clinical supervision.

BOX 5.3 | *Some alternative models of clinical supervision based on a lack of understanding*

■ The Road Works Model – telling supervisees which direction to take in practice

■ The Firefighter Model – dampening down the smouldering fires that flare up every now and then in practice

■ The Harbour Master Model – ensuring a place of safety in stormy practice waters

■ The Architect Model – getting in an expert to plan how to solve supervisee problems

■ The Clare Rayner Model – a cup of tea and a chat for disillusioned practitioners

■ The Exocet Model – seeking out individuals to destroy their confidence in practice (and make them leave)

■ The Great Pretender Model – avoiding confrontational issues by making out that everything is fine (and colluding with the bad bits of practice)

■ The 'Medical' Model – 'curing' supervisees of their practice ailments (but catching them yourself as the supervisor)

| BOX 5.4 | Roles and responsibilities in clinical supervision (reproduced by permission of Redbridge Healthcare NHS Trust Directorate of Nursing and Quality 1998) |

Clinical supervisees

- Holding my own record of the supervision session
- Being prepared for the supervision session, having identified issues to discuss
- Developing the ability to share these issues freely
- Identifying and talking about the kind of response that is useful to me
- Becoming more aware of my own organisational constraints and their implications and the organisational constraints on the supervisor
- Being open to feedback and using it to reflect future practice
- Developing the ability to discriminate what feedback is useful
- Noticing when I justify, explain or defend listening to feedback
- Implementing any action plan developed during supervision

Clinical supervisors

- Ensuring that privacy is available for the supervision session
- Helping the supervisee explore and clarify their own thinking, feelings and beliefs in order to become a reflective practitioner
- Giving clear and constructive feedback
- Sharing information, experiences and skills appropriately
- Challenging practice we see and agree action with supervisee to rectify deficits identified
- Being aware of the organisational constraints upon the supervisee
- Recording the attendance at the clinical supervision session
- Ending the supervision session

Shared responsibilities of the clinical supervisor and the clinical supervisee

- Arranging when and where the next session will take place
- Preparing for the supervision session to ensure time is used effectively
- Determining the frequency with which supervision occurs following the local guidelines
- Maintaining confidentiality
- Reviewing regularly the usefulness of supervision
- Knowing the boundaries of the supervision process and what responsibilities each has if the boundaries are infringed
- Informing the line manager of any cancellations of the supervision session

NB. The boundaries of confidentiality within clinical supervision are: anything that is illegal; breaches of the individual's Code of Conduct (UKCC 1992); or infringements of Redbridge Healthcare NHS Trust Disciplinary Policies.

BOX 5.5	Line manager roles and responsibilities (reproduced by permission of BHB Community NHS Trust–Nursing Directorate 1997)

- Ensuring adequate systems of support and supervision exist for staff they manage
- Incorporating clinical supervision into the development of individual personal development plans
- Monitoring that each health professional accesses clinical supervision with a designated clinical supervisor
- Monitoring the efficacy of clinical supervision within the area they are responsible for
- Assisting staff in managing time effectively so that they can participate in regular clinical supervision
- Negotiating with clinical supervisors the number of supervisees they can reasonably be expected to adopt
- Being responsible for dealing promptly and appropriately with issues arising out of clinical supervision that are brought to their attention by the supervisee or supervisor
- Consider the ongoing educational and training needs of clinical supervisors, e.g. briefings, updates and professional development
- Monitoring the uptake of clinical supervision by clinical supervisors

Line managers are important too, to legitimise clinical supervision in practice, and have their own roles and responsibilities (Box 5.5).

Obtaining agreement on how sessions will be organised

While it is relatively straightforward to adopt a 'shopping list' approach to organising supervision, more thought-provoking discussion will be generated by working out ways in which goals can actually be achieved. Most clinical supervision policies set out a framework within which clinical supervision can be operated in practice, but the specifics will need to be agreed between the participants during the first session. As stated earlier, developing the contract is an essential part of achieving rapport and understanding. It is also a way of beginning to put into operation the practicalities of regularly engaging in the process. Box 5.6 offers some signposts as to how to organise the first clinical supervision session.

Although they are seemingly straightforward enough, the key concept for both parties is that they should **agree** about rules and boundaries.

How participants will know if clinical supervision is working or not

Key statement 6 of the UKCC (1996) position statement on clinical supervision emphasises the need to evaluate the effectiveness of clinical supervision: 'Evaluation of clinical supervision is needed to assess how it influences care, practice standards and the service. Evaluation systems should be determined locally.'

| BOX 5.6 | *Some signposts for agreeing the organisation of clinical supervision sessions* |

The practicalities of supervision

- How often?
- Length of sessions?
- Where will it take place?
- Do any rooms need to be booked in advance?
- How can supervision fit in with existing responsibilities and workload?
- Are there good times for both parties?
- What is the procedure if a session has to be cancelled?
- What are reasonable/unreasonable grounds for cancelling?
- Is the environment conducive to being able to think about practice?
- How is confidentiality to be maintained?
- What happens in the event of not getting on with one another in supervision?
- Mutually agree a time in advance to review how clinical supervision is going

The content of supervisory sessions

- What individual expectations do you each have of one another?
- Who is responsible for setting the agenda and how will this be done?
- How will time be weighted towards the issues raised in supervision?
- What might be considered priority issues to discuss?
- Are you both clear about what you can talk about in sessions?
- What are acceptable ways of giving feedback to one another?
- What are unacceptable ways of giving feedback to one another?
- Is anything not acceptable to discuss in clinical supervision?
- When do personal issues obscure professional ones?

Session structure

- Prepare for the session by reminding yourself what went on previously
- The supervisor has a responsibility for ensuring a conducive environment
- Start the session on time
- Review what went on in the previous session and follow up issues where necessary
- Find out how each other is feeling before agreeing on a fresh agenda (it can be useful to know of any practice dramas that have occurred immediately before attending that might have an impact on the session)
- Prioritise the agenda
- The supervisee describes the issue(s) to the supervisor
- The supervisor listens and gives feedback to the supervisee
- Jointly analyse issues and work out ways together of moving forward
- The supervisor should summarise what has been happening in the session and clarify with the supervisee issues discussed and subsequent actions
- Record session as previously agreed
- The supervisor should ask the supervisee for feedback on supervisor performance
- Check date/time/venue for next session

BOX 5.7	*Provision of arrangements if a supervisory relationship breaks down (reproduced by permission of BHB Community NHS Trust–Nursing Directorate 1997)*

In the event that a supervisee wishes to change his/her clinical supervisor, he/she may do so, after giving the existing clinical supervisor clear reasons for doing so – either verbally or written. It is important that a rationale is given, as reasons for discontinuing clinical supervision are not always due to dissatisfaction. For example, the supervisee may have needs which may be met more appropriately by a clinical supervisor with a different professional background.

The clinical supervisor may advise the supervisee to access another clinical supervisor from a different discipline/speciality for particular issues/aspects of practice, while still remaining the clinical supervisor.

Where possible, any disagreements between a supervisee and supervisor should remain between the two parties involved and be resolved informally. The renegotiation of the supervisory contract may assist this process.

Where issues cannot be dealt with informally, such as claims of harassment or professional incompetence, the individual (either supervisee or supervisor) should inform the respective line manager, who will take appropriate action in accordance with Trust policy.

Monitoring the effectiveness of clinical supervision is dealt with in depth in Chapter 11, but establishing a contract in the early stages can form a baseline from which to gauge how sessions are going. It is very likely that, as most practitioners will be new to the process, misunderstandings will occur as part of the learning process. Many misunderstandings in clinical supervision are based on poor communication, which is the subject of Chapter 9. In some cases, a mismatching of supervisor and supervisee may occur. It is therefore important to have regular reviews, e.g. after six sessions, to monitor how both parties feel about the way the process is going.

Adopting a regular review of what is happening ensures that both the supervisee and the supervisor have a way of removing themselves from the situation other than by simply not turning up or cancelling sessions. Even not-so-good experiences in clinical supervision can be looked upon as valuable learning experiences for next time. Some clinical supervision policies cater for this eventuality, alongside any local arrangements made in the first session. An example can be found in Box 5.7.

In your opinion, for what reasons might the clinical supervisor advise the supervisee to seek another clinical supervisor? How might potential difficulties be dealt with in the contractual stage of clinical supervision?

Clinical supervision is not an exact science and there is currently a lack of information about how an effective clinical supervision session can be recognised, as well as how its effect in clinical care can be measured. One of the ways around this is to establish a habit of documenting what goes on. Keeping documentary evidence will probably be the responsibility of the supervisee, while the supervisor is responsible for the more basic record-keeping, e.g. the venue, date, time and parties involved. Despite this, record-keeping and documentation are often issues of concern for new supervisees.

METHODS OF RECORDING AND DOCUMENTING CLINICAL SUPERVISION

In my experience of working as a clinical supervisor, I have often had to deal during the first session with supervisee anxiety at the prospect of recording and documenting supervision sessions. As has already been described, the first session is important for working out ground rules and boundaries, including the importance of maintaining confidentiality. But this can seem at odds with the requirement for the supervisee to keep some form of formal documentation. How to keep records and documentation is an essential element of both supervisee and supervisor preparation and training, and is discussed in more detail in Chapters 6 and 7.

In what ways do you think keeping records or formalising documentation might be worrying for the supervisee?

In what ways do you think worries about documentation could be allayed by the clinical supervisor?

Clark et al (1998, p. 52) rightly suggest that neglecting this sort of anxiety-provoking issue can lead to misconceptions on the part of the supervisee, resulting, at best, in lip service only being paid to supervision and, at worst, in a complete refusal to participate. But documentation worries can also affect the supervisor. Without some initial discussion and a working agreement on confidentiality, Bond & Holland (1998, p. 91) suggest that both the supervisor and supervisee may be tempted not to keep any records at all. Brown & Bourne (1996, p. 65) refer to the supervisor's own potential insecurity while establishing the contract: 'Lacking confidence, [supervisors] may then unconsciously collude with unclear expectations and boundaries, because these confuse the supervisory relationship, and make their role more obscure … particularly where supervisors feel they are being caught up and overtaken by their supervisees.'

I remember that, as a new clinical supervisor, I also experienced such worries.

In reality, documentation is simply a description of what happened during the session, and subsequent reflections and actions. The supervisee is responsible for willingly disclosing information about their clinical practice and deciding (in the first session) how to record it. Clinical supervision is not an interrogation, and information about what happens in practice cannot be forced out of a supervisee by a supervisor.

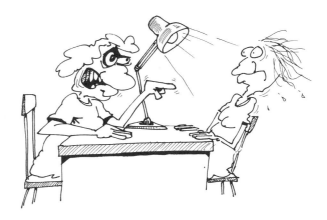

History Box

In my early supervision sessions I felt awkward and insecure about confronting a supervisee with the documentation issue so early in the establishment of the relationship, fearing that documentation was synonymous with managerial supervision. Because I did not do so, a situation arose at a later stage that was much more difficult to retrieve, caused by my not being able to remember what had happened in the last session 6 weeks earlier. The consequence for the supervisee was a lack of continuity at the start of each session and for me a feeling of guilt that the supervisee might think they were not important to me. It was impossible to recap what had happened before, as the supervisee had also failed to keep notes! I learned an important lesson about the necessity of getting access to regular supervision myself (as a supervisor).

What I also failed to appreciate were the possible consequences of not keeping records. For instance, what if I needed to show evidence to my educational line manager of the time I was spending on supervision as opposed to teaching? My own supervision helped me to learn not to feel that I was a bad role model, as I and the supervisee had both unwittingly contributed to the situation by our unwillingness to keep records. It was also an opportunity to show that I was not an expert in supervision but could learn from early mistakes and move on.

I changed supervisor recently because my previous supervisor had serious domestic problems and needed some space in which to recover. In my new contract, I negotiated that all sessions would be audiotaped. Now I can replay the sessions in the car some time after the event. I use a dictating machine to make a note of the important aspects. This forms the basis of my documentation, which I send to my supervisor before the next session so that we both have a record of what happened last time. This makes supervision more consistent and removes the worry of forgetting what was said – I often haven't got time to write up my supervision notes straight away. What has surprised me most is how much I must have forgotten about sessions with my previous supervisor, who preferred to operate without documentation other than the contract.

Similarly, you cannot force someone to reflect on their practice. Instead, there is an expectation that the supervisee and the supervisor (in their own supervision) will be equally committed to the process of sharing issues from clinical practice with the intention of enhancing it. The 'broad principles' approach to contracts usually also applies to clinical supervision records and documentation (Figures 5.2A–C). Such documentation is not just a record of poor practice and shortcomings, it is a personal and professional development learning tool.

While the agreed, written and signed contract is an essential part of clinical supervision, the status of ongoing record-keeping is less clear. Dimond (1998) considers a voluntary system of clinical supervision to be one where a contractual requirement is not demanded but the arrangement rests instead on the willing offer of one to be supervised and the other to supervise. Most cases of clinical supervision are likely to be of this type. Although such a system is open to non-participation on the part of practitioners who would really benefit from clinical supervision, they are still professionally accountable for their practice.

The current stance taken by the UKCC (1996, Neal 1998), which has not been tested in a court of law, is that if an employer includes in the contract of employment a requirement that the employee undertakes clinical supervision,

Figure 5.2A   *An example of a clinical supervision record used in practice*

HOSPITALS

CONFIDENTIAL JOINT RECORD OF CLINICAL SUPERVISION

Date: ....   Time: ....

Name of supervisee/or description of group

Session number

Name of supervisor

Reiteration Clinical Supervision ground rules
Discussed: YES/NO
Comments:

SUMMARY OF SESSION:

Key issues covered

Action being carried out

Issues to be followed up at next session

DATE OF NEXT CLINICAL SUPERVISION SESSION

Date: ....   Time: ....

Venue: ....

then the documentation is the property of the employer. However, if an employer merely encourages an employee to participate in clinical supervision, then any records made *are probably* the property of the employer. In both cases, the content of clinical supervision records is clearly the province of the participants and depends on what was disclosed at the time. Keeping records

Figure 5.2B	*An example of a clinical supervision record used in practice*

CLINICAL SUPERVISION DOCUMENTATION

Faculty of Health

<u>TO BE COMPLETED AND KEPT BY THE CLINICAL SUPERVISEE:</u>

Date: Time: Venue:

Supervisor:

Supervisee:

ISSUES/ACTIONS RAISED IN LAST SESSION:

Main learning for supervisee:

ISSUES BROUGHT TO THIS SESSION BY SUPERVISEE:

SUPERVISEE ACTIONS REQUIRED FOR NEXT SESSION:

is therefore an important safeguard because they can be presented at the next session as an accurate account by all parties of what went on during the previous meeting.

Two sorts of record have been described in this chapter: a contractual record agreeing how clinical supervision will be organised and ongoing documentation

Figure 5.2C   *An example of a clinical supervision record used in practice*

Forest Healthcare Trust Mental Health Directorate
CS1 – Clinical Supervision Policy
April 1999

RECORD OF SUPERVISION

Date: Name of Supervisee:

Time: Name of Supervisor:

Venue:

Session Number: Date of Next Session: Date:

Time:

Venue:

Reflection on last session:

Issues brought to supervision:

Issues for reflection/action:

that describes what happened during a session. Both are intended to promote safe practice as well as safe supervisory practice. While the formal contract is essential to clarify how clinical supervision is organised, the ongoing documentation is developmental for both the supervisor and the supervisee and can even form the basis for further reflection to maintain professional registration

(Ham Ying 1996, UKCC 1997). These records will probably also provide evidence for evaluating the effectiveness (or not) of clinical supervision in practice and also provide the necessary individual evidence to the organisation of participating in clinical governance (Butterworth & Woods 1999).

On reflection ... chapter summary

What are the key elements of this chapter?

- All parties engaged in clinical supervision have individual roles and responsibilities as well as shared ones
- A clinical supervision contract can make what goes on more explicit
- Drawing up a contract together in clinical supervision can share the ownership of it
- All parties require adequate preparation to contribute to the drawing up of the contract
- It can be useful to identify what clinical supervision is not before embarking on clinical supervision itself
- Some aspects of supervision structure and content need to be agreed beforehand
- Recording and documenting sessions can help bridge the time between sessions and help to measure the effectiveness of supervision in practice

So what difference does this make to the way I am operating my clinical/supervisory practice?

Now what actions will need to be taken as a result of my reflections?

REFERENCES

Bailey D 1987 Guidance in open learning: a manual of practice. National Institute for Careers in Education and Counselling, Manpower Services Commission, London

Bond M, Holland S 1998 Skills of clinical supervision for nurses. Open University Press, Buckingham

Brown A, Bourne I 1996 The social work supervisor. Open University Press, Milton Keynes

Butterworth T, Woods D 1999 Clinical governance and Clinical Supervision: working together to ensure safe and accountable practice. A Briefing Paper University of Manchester UK

Clark A, Dooher J, Fowler J, Phillips A, North R, Wells A 1998 Implementing clinical supervision. In: Fowler J (ed) The handbook of clinical supervision – your questions answered. Quay Books, Salisbury, ch 2

Dimond B 1998 Legal aspects of clinical supervision 1: Employer vs employee. British Journal of Nursing 7(7): 393–395

Dolley J, Davies C, Murray P 1998 Clinical supervision a development pack for nurses (K509). Open University Press, Buckingham

Gadd D, Mahood N 1995 Clinical supervision – a time for professional development.

Cartmel NDU (Mental Health Services of Salford), Salford

Ham Ying S 1996 Not up to standard. Nursing Times 92(15): 28–30

Morrison T 1996 Staff supervision in social care. Pavilion, Brighton

Neal K 1998 A framework for managing risk. Nursing Times Learning Curve 1(12): 4–5

Power S 1999 Nursing Supervision: a guide for clinical practice Sage, London, UK

UKCC 1992 Code of professional conduct. United Kingdom Central Council for Nursing, Midwifery and Health Visiting, London

UKCC 1996 Position statement on clinical supervision for nursing and health visiting. United Kingdom Central Council for Nursing, Midwifery and Health Visiting, London

UKCC 1997 PREP and you. United Kingdom Central Council for Nursing, Midwifery and Health Visiting, London

West Midlands Clinical Supervision Learning Set (1998) Clinical Supervision: Getting it right in your organisation. A critical guide to good practice. West Midlands Clinical Supervision Learning Set, c/o School of Health Sciences, University of Birmingham, UK

6

Essential skills for clinical supervisees

INTRODUCTION

Much of the contemporary literature on clinical supervision in nursing has tended towards the development of the clinical supervisor at the expense of the supervisee. Is it any surprise that Sams (1997, p. 44), in her evaluation of implementing clinical supervision, found that, despite an infrastructure being put in place, supervisees did not take it up?

Supervisees are not passive players in the clinical supervision process but are central to its success (Bond & Holland 1998, p. 81). In my experience of good and not so good supervision sessions, the old adage 'you only get out what you put in' comes to mind. Although this is applicable to both parties in clinical supervision, a motivated and interested supervisee can really push the process forward, often resulting in marked changes in their clinical practice.

It is worth considering the 'Doomsday scenario' for clinical supervision, if supervisees are not committed to having regular clinical supervision in practice or actively seeking it out. In this instance organisations have three choices:

- Continue to persevere with the slow uptake of clinical supervision in the practice area by increasing supervisees' training time and continuing to 'wait and see'

- Become disillusioned with the slow uptake and begin to dismantle the supervisory infrastructures already put into place
- Insist that clinical supervision is such a good idea for clinical practice, according to whatever agenda, that it is made mandatory for all qualified staff in practice, thus 'kick starting' the process

In the longer term, preparation of clinical supervisees needs to become embedded in preregistration nurse education, where the continuum of supervision really begins, as outlined in an earlier chapter. In this way, following a period of preceptorship, clinical supervision will be expected, as a continuation of lifelong learning in nursing. It is interesting to speculate as to whether the students of today expect to be the supervisees and subsequently the supervisors of tomorrow.

This chapter directly addresses clinical supervisees, who often begin supervision expecting the clinical supervisor to be skilled in what *they* do, rather than in developing the supervisee's own skills. By 'skills' is meant here the ability to maximise the use of the time available in a session. At the end of the chapter is a supervisee self-assessment that can be used as a baseline to measure the effectiveness of individual supervisee performance in clinical supervision.

CLINICAL SUPERVISION AS STORYTELLING

A metaphor is concerned with the transference of meaning from one situation to another (Froggatt 1998). Storytelling by the supervisee, I would suggest, is a useful metaphor for the whole process of clinical supervision. Most stories have a beginning, middle and end and the structure of a clinical supervision session could, metaphorically speaking, embody the telling of a story about clinical practice.

Vezeau (1993, p. 193) illustrates the value of storytelling in paediatric nursing and how talking about the human, feeling aspects of an experience can develop a closer relationship between the supervisee and the supervisor: 'Reading a journal article or a textbook, we do not become personally attached to the information or appreciate what the experience is truly like ... all stories are relational, involving storyteller, audience and the story as vehicle, narrative is a partnership requiring openness and involvement'.

Bowles (1995) was surprised by the lack of references to storytelling in the UK nursing literature. He maintains that British nurses often tell stories in critical incident reviews, reflective journals, professional portfolios and clinical supervision relationships but do not seem to realise that they are storytelling! Perhaps the term 'storytelling' fits better in a clinical supervision context because it is not predominantly an 'academic' pursuit.

The importance of the ability to tell a story as a supervisee skill in clinical supervision is the active element played out by the supervisee in telling the story to the clinical supervisor. The clinical supervisor pays attention to the story but should be careful not to get too wrapped up in the content. The essence of a good story is in how it is told; the clinical supervisor then helps the supervisee to derive meaning and see the bigger issues that emerge from it. Preparing for clinical supervision as a supervisee can also be fitted in to the storytelling metaphor if one examines the anatomy of a clinical supervision session again.

THE ANATOMY OF A CLINICAL SUPERVISION SESSION

Breaking down the clinical supervision session into parts offers a basic structure for supervisee storytelling (Box 6.1).

More importantly, it demonstrates the active role and skills required of the supervisee to enhance the clinical supervision encounter – the skill not just to prepare to tell an interesting story but not to allow the clinical supervisor to put the book down. It is important to remember that the structure outlined does not include the first contractual session, described in Chapter 5, in which emphasis is necessarily more on producing results. You may wish to add to the box other points that seem important to you, drawn from your supervisee training or preparatory workshops.

IDENTIFYING SKILLS TRANSFERABLE FROM CLINICAL PRACTICE THAT COULD BE USED BY A SUPERVISEE

It is probably obvious from Box 6.1 that as a practitioner you already have some experience of listening to stories as well as telling them – e.g. finding out about a patient/person's background in order to be able to plan care, telling relatives about a family member's progress, exchanging practice stories during handover.

What skills could a supervisee possibly transfer to the supervision situation from clinical practice? Had you even considered that a supervisee needed any skills at all in supervision? You may wish to compare some of your own ideas to my list in Box 6.2, which is based on the anatomy of a clinical supervision session.

The range of transferable skills might have surprised you. Many of them you may not even have noticed, or not have recognised as useful to a supervisee in clinical supervision. Engaging in clinical supervision requires a positive approach and an open mind on how it might enhance your clinical practice. The following comments are not unusual in clinical supervisee workshops:

The time I'm spending in clinical supervision could be better spent with my patients.

I don't need supervision – I don't have any problems and I'm a senior staff member.

I'm not going to supervision to be grilled on my practice.... I've not been disciplined yet in 3 years as a staff nurse.

Clearly, supervisees new to supervision are naturally going to be anxious about exposing their clinical practice to another person for critical review. It can be useful to remind practitioners that clinical supervision is different from supervised practice, with which they will be more familiar and which, of course, includes some form of assessment. Bishop (1998), as cited in the opening chapter, describes the 'what' and 'why' of clinical supervision, which can help clarify the supervisee's role (Box 6. 3).

| BOX 6.1 | *The anatomy of a clinical supervision session from a storyteller's point of view* |

Adequately prepare for storytelling beforehand

■ Review documentation for any previous session

■ Think about what you want to discuss and make a note of it, or tape-record the session (with the supervisor's permission beforehand)

■ Give yourself plenty of time to get to the venue

■ Plan your day beforehand/warn others that you will need to leave work temporarily

■ Other points?

Opening the practice story

■ Review what went on in the previous session and check that the supervisor understands it

■ Check how you are feeling as the storyteller (e.g. are you tired or is something happening that is likely to limit your storytelling ability?)

■ Try to identify beforehand the practice stories you most wish to talk about

■ Work out with the supervisor what practice story(ies) you want to tell in the limited time you have together

■ Other points?

Telling the practice story

■ Try to give a full description of what happened, using your own words and metaphors to illustrate the situation

■ Use the opportunity to take the lead – it is your story and your clinical supervision session

■ Be willing and open enough to consider different endings to your practice story

■ Record or document any alternative ways of ending the practice story

■ Other points?

Audience reaction to your practice story

■ As you tell the story, consider the reaction to what happened of some of the main characters in your story other than just yourself

■ Jointly check for understanding of the practice story told

■ Listen to the supervisor's precis of your practice story; has the supervisor fully understood?

■ Jointly agree with the supervisor any alternative ways there might have been to end the practice story

■ Agree on any plan of action to take into future practice situations

■ Record the story in the way agreed during the initial contractual session

■ Offer positive feedback to the audience (supervisor) for listening to your story

■ Check date/time/venue for next session

■ Other points?

BOX 6.2	*Some transferable supervisee skills from clinical practice*
Anatomy of a supervision session (from Box .6.1)	**Transferable practice skills that can be used by the supervisee**
Adequately preparing for practice storytelling beforehand	Record keeping Care planning Personal time management Liaising with colleagues
Opening the practice story	Picking up cues for patient/client understanding Recognising how practitioner performance can be related to how you are feeling on the day Prioritising what clinical practice is important to hand over to colleagues Working within time constraints
Telling the practice story	Being accountable for what you do as a practitioner Being open to considering different ways of caring for patient/client while doing it Able to recognise and report to significant others changes in the patient's condition/client's circumstances
Audience reaction to your story	Able to recognise others' needs before your own Able to listen to other people's concerns Regularly finding out more from others about unfamiliar situations Able to adapt to different situations that arise in clinical practice

Supervisees should be encouraged to prepare for what is brought to and discussed in supervision. In this way, they will begin to make more effective use of the time that clinical supervision offers for formal reflective practice.

Consider Wendy, a community nurse supervisee who commented at the end of her first clinical supervision encounter:

> Do you know, I feel really positive about clinical supervision now.... I hadn't realised that it was really for me.... I thought that clinical supervision was something my manager wanted me to take up because she was concerned about my new role in clinical practice.... I'll start to look out now for some of the ordinary things that happen in my practice to bring to supervision to help you understand what I get up to as stroke liaison nurse.... Thanks for some of the ideas you gave me for taking charge of my own supervision.... I'll let others know about it so they can think about taking up clinical supervision.

This is very different from unskilled supervisees who expect to be dragged kicking and screaming into clinical supervision.

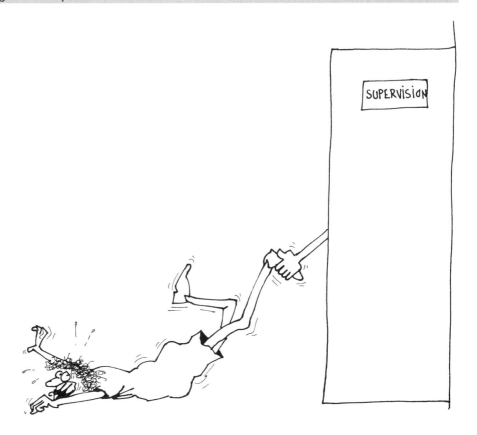

BOX 6.3	*The 'what' and 'why' of clinical supervision (Bishop 1998)*

The 'what' of clinical supervision:

'Clinical supervision is a designated interaction between two or more practitioners, within a safe and supportive environment, which enables a continuum of reflective, critical analysis of care, to ensure quality patient services' (Bishop 1998, p. 8).

The 'why' of clinical supervision

- To safeguard standards of practice
- To develop the individual both professionally and personally
- To promote excellence in nursing care (Bishop 1998, p. 12).

SIX ESSENTIAL SKILLS OF A CLINICAL SUPERVISEE

Despite all the hype surrounding clinical supervision, there is not, as yet, any agreed way of doing it in nursing, and why should there be? A range of approaches to clinical supervision are explored in Chapter 8. While practitioners often seek a right way of doing things, clinical supervision requires the establishment of principles and the exercising of some autonomy as to how these are to be achieved. The previous chapter examined how the first meeting is an important part of negotiating as a supervisee what seems to you to be appropriate for your own practice.

All parties in clinical supervision have more than enough skills between them to make it work; it just requires a commitment to wanting to explore practice on a regular basis, in time that is protected and legitimised by the organisation. Clinical supervision is simply extending some of the skills you already use in nursing practice to improve it, not something imposed by those outside. Clearly, different specialisms in nursing require different skills. This is why a range of clinical supervision schemes needs to be developed from within practice, guided by principles negotiated with the supervisee.

It is important as a supervisee to begin to be aware of what kinds of thing go well and not so well in clinical supervision. In this way, the myths about 'going for supervision' will be replaced by more accurate accounts of what really happens, and a body of supervision knowledge will begin to emerge from within clinical practice areas.

Six essential skills are necessary for the supervisee to develop to experience effective clinical supervision (Box 6.4).

BOX 6.4	Six skills essential to the supervisee for effective clinical supervision

- Make the session work for you, not just the supervisor
- Identify pertinent stories to disclose in the session
- Start to be aware of your 'self' in clinical practice
- Be open to receiving feedback on clinical performance
- Write as well as talk about practice stories
- Adopt a more proactive approach to practice 'problems'

Although seemingly mundane and glaringly obvious, it is unlikely that every supervisee will be competent in them all at first. Much will depend on the supervisory experience derived from the style or approach adopted together and is developed further in Chapter 8.

Essential skill 1: Make the session work for you, not just the supervisor

Nursing is essentially a personal as well as a social activity: the development of interpersonal relationships lies at the heart of all that nurses do. The clinical supervision relationship is no different. The key to a successful supervisory partnership lies in being open in the first meeting with the clinical supervisor to how clinical supervision can work for you as the supervisee. The participants have different roles and responsibilities, as discussed in Chapter 5. An important element will be developing the confidence to become more 'selfish' about what happens in *your* clinical supervision.

Adopting a more 'selfish' approach *before* engaging in clinical supervision can include getting more information about how it can work for you by:

- attending local study days or workshops
- speaking to a course tutor at the local college
- obtaining your own position statement on clinical supervision, or chatting to the responsible professional officer at the UKCC
- speaking to your line manager, who will know of local developments
- talking to colleagues already in supervision about what goes on
- chatting informally with an established clinical supervisor
- obtaining a copy of any local clinical supervision policy or protocols
- networking with similar practitioners in other organisations about how it works for them
- asking the college librarian to help you do a literature search on clinical supervision, or visiting a relevant web site
- obtaining some articles to discuss in your practice area.

If you do not know what to expect, or what the purpose of clinical supervision is, how can you be in control of what happens in the sessions? If you begin clinical supervision with an idea of how you intend using it to help you with your clinical practice, this places you at the centre of clinical supervision as the supervisee.

Perhaps you being at the centre does not happen all that often in your practice area? Your voice is not somehow loud enough or considered important enough to really make a difference, perhaps? In clinical supervision, you have a choice to continue with the current situation or move towards something better. The clinical supervision encounter is a way of placing you at the centre of your practice, as well as giving you some ideas of how to reach what you see as important goals.

The relationship you have or develop with your clinical supervisor will obviously be crucial to all of this. If you are unhappy with the way things are going in supervision, negotiate a change in your contract, or change your supervisor! It really is better to start clinical supervision by having some informed idea at the beginning of what you want, and agree with your supervisor on this. You can then begin as a supervisee to explore ways through your practice stories to move towards what you consider good practice to be.

If you have not started clinical supervision yet:
You probably already have an idea of what engaging in clinical supervision means, otherwise you would not be interested enough to read this book. Write your own clinical supervision story, or divide an A4 sheet of paper into two halves. On one of the halves jot down what, as a supervisee, you would like your clinical supervision to be like. What sorts of thing would it include? On the other half do the opposite: jot down what, as a supervisee, you would not like your clinical supervision to be like. What sorts of thing would it not include? If you actively engage in this, you will begin to understand the clinical supervision experience. You are able to take time out to be 'selfish' about what you want to happen, while having an idea of what you need to look out for that will tell you that clinical supervision isn't working for you.

If you have already started clinical supervision:
You already know what engaging in clinical supervision as a clinical supervisee means to you. Write your own clinical supervision story, or divide an A4 sheet of paper into two halves. On one of the halves jot down what, as a supervisee, you like about your clinical supervision. What sorts of thing does this include? On the other half do the opposite: jot down what you dislike most about your clinical supervision at present. What sorts of thing does it not include or what sorts of thing does it include that you do not like? If you actively engage in this, you are in a position to turn around your clinical supervision if you are really unhappy with it. Why have you not already taken time out before this to be more 'selfish' about getting what you really want out of your supervision time?

Essential skill 2: Identify pertinent stories to disclose in the session

It has already been suggested that the supervisee's practice story(ies) will form the basis of the clinical supervision session. An essential skill for the supervisee is in deciding which stories are important. This is not always straightforward, for a number of reasons:

- Not making a note of significant things that have happened in practice since the last supervision session
- Using informal chats in practice as a substitute for supervision
- Not being used to reflecting on your practice with others in any depth
- Not realising that a particular story is worth exploring
- Being unwilling or anxious about exposing a particular aspect of your clinical practice
- Not being in control of clinical supervision.

Many of the above can occur because you don't give yourself enough preparation time between supervision sessions. Sometimes this preparation will need to be done away from the pressured work environment. Inadequate preparation will mean that a large proportion of clinical supervision time is spent mulling over past events to discuss, which can become boring and be difficult for either party to sustain for any length of time. Supervision time can be better spent if you have already given some thought to different ways of developing issues that have emerged. In this way the process will inform and enhance your clinical practice.

Keeping a written record, rather than simply a mental note of issues that crop up in clinical practice, is useful and need not be time-consuming. It could simply take the form of a collection of 'tabloid newspaper banner headlines' that you collect over time to remind you of what went on. Thinking of the headline to match the story will also reinforce your memory of it, and help identify what is important about it for you, so that you can bring it up in the next supervision session.

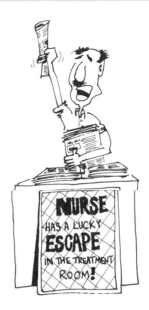

Not all supervision time will be spent in relating new practice stories. The early part of the session is likely to be taken up with reflecting upon how you have managed (or not) with something that came up in the last session. If you are unable to think of something to talk about in a supervision session (which is very unlikely), you might instead wish to consider completing some of the sentences in Box 6.5 at the end of a shift.

BOX 6.5	*Some ideas for things to take to clinical supervision*

Complete any of the following after you have finished your shift:

■ Something that went well for me today was …

■ I really felt like a nurse today because …

■ What really drove me mad today was …

■ What I attempted to do in this situation was …

■ Something that bothers me about what I do is …

■ I really think I need more information about …

■ What really puzzled me today was …

■ If I had the chance to do that again I would …

■ I felt really stupid about …

Notice that not all of the ideas in Box 6.5 are negative ones: some record positive practice experiences as well. Clinical supervision will become a very negative experience and only serve to demoralise the supervisee if the focus is always on the down side of practice. It can be quite enlightening to recall something that you were pleased about. The focus can then be: 'In what way did you think this was good? What did you say or do?' Exploring why something was successful can be a major source of learning as the supervisee begins to understand the answer to the question and tries to repeat the good practice.

Confidentiality in the supervisory partnership is essential and it will take time, as the supervisory relationship develops, before you feel comfortable enough to begin to disclose some aspects of your practice. 'Will the supervisor laugh at me or be shocked?' and 'What will happen if the supervisor lets this out to my manager?' are not uncommon supervisee anxieties. Listen out for supervisor disclosures, e.g. that she/he feels a bit nervous in his/her new role as clinical supervisor, that indicate that the supervisor is also becoming more comfortable and more open with you.

You, the supervisee, have an equal responsibility to keep what goes on in the session confidential. It is as important that what you thought of a supervisor's performance is not discussed in the coffee room as what you suspect the supervisor thinks about your performance as a practitioner! Fear of a lack of confidentiality in the clinical supervision relationship requires urgent discussion, perhaps with a third party, as it obviously means that important stories may be withheld from clinical supervision.

Essential skill 3: Start to be aware of your 'self' in clinical practice

History Box	I often recount the story of how a junior student was once talking to me about a clinical placement in the Accident & Emergency Department. She was very excited because she had found an area of nursing that she felt she wanted to make her career. One of the staff nurses she was working with was, the student said, 'brilliant'. When I probed a bit further, the student gave a number of examples of how this staff nurse 'always got lumbered with breaking bad news' because she was 'so good, the way she dealt with such tricky situations'. I suggested that, next time she was on placement, the student asked the staff nurse how she had become so good at her job, as she had obviously made such an impact on the student's practice.
	When I next saw the student she said she had asked the staff nurse how she had become so good at Accident & Emergency work. The staff nurse's response had been to go very red at the thought that someone had noticed the way she practised and to reply, 'It's nothing special, just routine!'

Beginning to notice your 'self' in clinical practice does not always require the help of a clinical supervisor. In this case, a student had 'noticed' and wanted to emulate what, for her, was such an excellent role model. The trouble was that the staff nurse was unaware of what she was doing, let alone being able to articulate it when somebody told her that they had noticed it! It can be very difficult for practitioners who are used to 'giving themselves' to really notice 'themselves' more actively during busy clinical practice. Clinical supervision offers an opportunity for the supervisee to begin this 'noticing' process and facilitating this is an important function of the clinical supervisor (Chapters 8 and 9).

Morrison & Burnard (1991, p. 130) consider the self as being composed of three integrated domains: the thinking, feeling and behaving self (Figure 6.1).

| **Figure 6.1** | *Three aspects of the self (integrated circles)* |

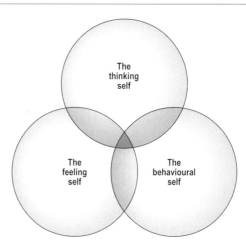

Thinking is a mental process that covers such things as ideas, how to solve problems and the consideration of different viewpoints. Feeling involves the emotional aspects of the self, while behaving describes what we do.

New & Cormack (1997, p. 25), in a book exploring the motives and behaviours of individuals, begin with the question 'Why did I do that?', to explore these three different aspects of the self. It is also a useful model to consider in clinical supervision to help supervisees notice more about 'themselves' in clinical practice. The three aspects of the self can be visualised as a garden water butt (Figure 6.2).

The clinical practice *situation* triggers the *thoughts* of the practitioner, which trigger the *feelings* of the practitioner, which result in the *behaviour* of the practitioner, or their observable actions. At the bottom of the water butt is the tap, which is opened by the supervisor to allow the supervisee story to drip through.

| **Figure 6.2** | *The three levels of the self* |

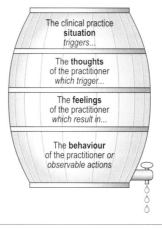

What usually drips through, or is often presented in a clinical supervision session, are the behaviours of the supervisee recounted in the practice story.

Draining the water butt in clinical supervision?
What will happen if the tap does not get turned on and off, but is kept running to drain the contents of the butt? We can do this by asking New & Cormack's question 'Why did I do that?'

- Imagine that reading this book is the **behaviour**, the observable action.
- What were the **feelings** you had immediately prior to picking up and reading this book?
- What **thoughts** triggered the feelings – can you recall them?
- Was there a **situation** in which you found yourself that made you **think** that reading this book (the **behaviour**) was a good idea? What are your **feelings** about reading the book now?

Although confusing at first, this exercise is a good illustration of the different facets of your 'self' at work, starting with a pretty simple example – reading the book in front of you. What you have been exposed to in this example is a rather simple method of enhancing your self-awareness, what Morrison & Burnard (1991, p. 141) refer to as: 'the process of noticing what we are doing or self monitoring. All that is involved is that you stay conscious of what you are doing, as you do it. In other words that you "stay awake" and develop the skill of keeping your attention focused on your actions, both verbal and nonverbal.'

Clearly, it is not possible to notice all of our actions and behaviours all of the time. Clinical supervision is an intentional activity in which the supervisee can begin to become more aware of the 'self' operating in clinical practice and choose between different actions on the basis of previous ones – what Heron (1973) refers to as 'the conscious use of the self'.

Read the account in the History Box of Hayley, a staff nurse supervisee in clinical supervision. Imagine you are the supervisor: what sorts of thing do you notice from this brief practice story that might help the supervisee notice her 'self' in clinical practice?

History Box   One thing that really winds me up is when, after slogging your guts out since early morning, the junior doctors arrive on the ward expecting me to run round after them so they look OK when the consultant does her ward round. If that's not bad enough, they didn't even have the courtesy to talk to Mrs Bloxham about her operation. She was worried sick ... I know, I've had to pick up the pieces ever since the anaesthetist didn't give her a full explanation about her temporary colostomy. Anyway, when I eventually got to the ward round – they had started without me – I realised that a male patient opposite was peeking through the only partially pulled curtains when they were checking her bag.... At that point I really flipped!

That ward sister wants me to apologise to the consultant next time she is on the ward.

What is Hayley's **behaviour** (actions) in this case?
- The behaviour associated with 'flipping' at the ward round, e.g. getting angry, raising her voice to other staff in front of the patient.

What were Hayley's **feelings** that led to the **behaviour**?
- Annoyance at the ward round having started without her and at the male patient peeking through the partially open bed curtains.

What **thoughts** of Hayley's were likely to have triggered the **feelings**?
- Not believing that the work she had done with Mrs Bloxham was valued by medical colleagues or peers, thinking that the doctors made use of her so they looked OK when the consultant came to the ward.

What **situation** is likely to have triggered the whole event?
- Noticing the male patient peeking in through the only partially closed curtains and having previously developed a close relationship with Mrs Bloxham and wanting to protect her dignity.

If you were Hayley's clinical supervisor, how could you help Hayley to begin to use her 'self' more consciously in future? Should she apologise?

Noticing the 'self' in clinical supervision is an intentional activity initiated by the supervisee. Although the clinical supervisor can encourage this, he/she is not able to prescribe it. In my view, one of the biggest challenges for the clinical supervisee is to not only notice the self from the comfort of the supervision armchair, but to put some of what is noticed back into clinical practice. For Hayley to action what has been noticed by the clinical supervisor will require her to be open to feedback on her clinical practice story told.

Essential skill 4: Be open to receiving feedback on clinical performance

As with many of the skills of the supervisee, being open to receiving feedback on clinical performance may seem obvious. However, this can be troubling not just for supervisees, but for supervisors as well, particularly if the supervisor has known the supervisee for some time. This dilemma is elaborated upon in Chapter 9. On the other hand, supervisees, having told their practice story, may feel embarrassed, away from the pressured situation, about how they acted. In other words, they may not be in the mood for any feedback.

McEvoy (1993) maintains that, before clinical supervision was introduced, many nurses felt that they were only told when what they did was not up to scratch and were given little positive feedback on their overall performance. This is likely to be so in Hayley's case – the ward sister is perhaps not fully aware of all the circumstances leading up to Hayley's behaviour, only of its immediate consequences.

Clinical supervision is different, in that the supervisor expects to give the supervisee more constructive feedback on their practice story. Clinical supervisees require feedback not just about performance that could be improved but about what was performed well, in order to maintain morale and reinforce that performance. In other words, the giving and receiving of feedback can be positive as well as negative. In Hayley's example, the supervisor might give feedback on the incident directly, or might wait for Hayley to ask for it. If she required positive feedback from the supervisor on her practice story she might ask:

What do you think was good about the way I acted in this situation?

Alternatively, Hayley could actively seek out negative feedback, having been aware of the supervisor's body language in response to her story:

I noticed you seem a bit surprised by what I said – do you think there were different ways of handling that situation better?

Good practice points for receiving feedback effectively

Negative feedback is not failure. Failures are another way of describing something you did not anticipate and did not want to happen. Feedback is an opportunity to learn from something you had not noticed but the clinical supervisor did. Based on Seijo's work on giving effective feedback (Seijo 1996, p. 53), here are some guidelines for Hayley to follow, based on the story in the History Box.

- Ask for feedback in a way that gives reassurance to the supervisor that you will not be offended if views are expressed openly:

  Hayley: I think you were a bit surprised with me that I lost my cool on the ward round – that's OK: tell me what you honestly think. I won't be offended and it will help me to consider not jumping straight in next time.

- Listen carefully to what is said by the supervisor, although you may feel uncomfortable. Resist the temptation to argue, explain or disagree.

  Hayley: Yes, but you don't understand....

  Supervisor: Hang on a minute, Hayley, let me have my say. I've listened to your practice story and I'm now trying to help you notice what I've noticed.

- Clarify what the supervisor is saying to you by asking questions after the feedback has been given.

  Hayley: Yes, but you don't understand. I had developed a close relationship with Mrs Bloxham – I like her a lot.

  Supervisor: I realise how special the patient was to you, Hayley, but perhaps in this instance it clouded your judgement on how to proceed.... Could you not have simply pulled the curtains properly around the bed while the examination was taking place?

  Hayley: Well I would have done if I had been on the ward at the time the round started, but … I had popped outside for a cigarette.

  Supervisor: Surely with your experience on this ward, Hayley, you had a pretty good idea of when the round would start, or could have asked someone to call you when they reached your named patients?

- Ask for suggestions about alternative ways of behaving.

  Hayley: I really do resent being the one who runs round for the junior doctors when I'm busy.

  Supervisor: Then why don't you stop running around after them, then?

  Hayley: Well, they need someone to support them, really.

  Supervisor: Well, why does it have to be you? Perhaps they have become dependent on you, and all the while it is you who could do with some support at this time ... have you spoken to Sister about what is happening?

- Take some time to decide whether you wish to act on the information.

  Supervisor: Perhaps you need to become more assertive rather than dealing with difficult situations in such an aggressive manner....

  Hayley: What do you mean, I'm aggressive! I'm one of the most ... sorry, I'm even starting it with you now.

  Supervisor: Don't apologise ... supervision is beginning to help you notice yourself. Are you aware of what being assertive means? It can be a useful leadership skill.

  Hayley: I think I need to chat with some more experienced colleagues and find out a bit more about the differences between being assertive and being aggressive ... I really want to get the vacant senior staff nurse post this year.

- Thank the supervisor for responding openly to your request for feedback. It may not have been easy.

  Hayley: Thanks for not biting my head off ... I really want to change my behaviour ... I'm beginning to see how clinical supervision can reflect what goes on in my clinical practice and yet I'm in a next-door building well away from my ward.

  Supervisor: I'm glad you are making so much progress, Hayley, but I did become a bit worried you might get stuck in to me verbally ... Just joking!

Essential skill 5: Write as well as talk about practice stories

A cursory glance at the latest lists of popular books is very likely to turn up, among the best-selling titles, a number of autobiographies of people who have painstakingly kept written records of what they did, or did not do, all through their careers. Imagine if nurses were to abandon the oral tradition in favour of a written tradition. Perhaps it is already happening.

Historically, nursing has been taught on the premise that there is a right way to go about it. Not surprisingly, when confronted with writing a reflective diary for the first time supervisees invariably require some reassurance they are doing it the right way. Street (1995, p. 148) suggests that beginning to write about one's clinical practice involves overcoming the hurdles not only of finding the time and describing our thoughts, feelings and behaviour in written form, but also of the sneaking suspicion that the effort may not really be worthwhile.

The discipline of writing is related to noticing the 'self' in practice in that, as discussed earlier, it turns an often unconscious practice activity into a deliberate and conscious act. In clinical supervision, 'freezing the action' (Street 1995, p. 151) by writing about practice will help the supervisee as well as the clinical supervisor to examine practice from a number of different perspectives.

Keeping a written journal as an aid to storytelling is a skill required of the supervisee. The association between keeping a reflective journal/log and clinical supervision is becoming more prominent within the UK nursing literature (Butcher 1995, Marrow et al 1997, Johns & Freshwater 1998). At the very least, the UKCC (1996, 1997) advocates that supervision records are kept, with many organisations now agreeing that the supervisee should keeps them within their professional portfolio as evidence for maintaining professional registration as well as to maintain confidentiality.

Essential skill 6: Adopt a more proactive approach to practice 'problems'

Although clinical supervision does not only have to be about supervisee 'problems', invariably the sessions start out like that. This may demonstrate the particular level that new supervisees are at, or the fact that supervisees in nursing practice value this approach the most. It is interesting when I challenge the supervisee to bring in something that went well for a change. This is, not surprisingly, more challenging for the supervisee, often used to adopting a 'problem'-orientated approach to clinical care using the nursing process. Although one of the first reflective tools in nursing, this tends to get stuck at identifying 'nursing' problems rather than 'patient' problems and is often viewed as a chore to be done during a busy shift rather than a meaningful account of how such 'problems' were solved.

The same approach, I have noticed, is adopted by inexperienced supervisees in clinical supervision. Often the problems they wish to bring to supervision are not really theirs but are complex and often intractable organisational dilemmas. It is difficult then to identify the supervisee's position within the story or to expect the supervisee to walk away from the session having personally achieved something from the discussion. Doing this can be a ploy on the part of the supervisee aimed at getting personally lost in complicated scenarios that protect them from having to disclose or expose their clinical practice 'self'. More usually, they have been indoctrinated into a reactive problem-centred approach to giving care, rather than adopting a more proactive solution-centred attitude.

While clinical supervision is not therapy, it can have therapeutic effects on the supervisee – having someone to bounce ideas around with in confidence, having an experienced practitioner to listen to you without judging you and to offer constructive support during a difficult period. Traditional models of psychiatry or psychotherapy, however, also tend to focus on the client's 'problems', exploring the past in some detail to help develop insight into why a 'problem' emerged and to help clients understand why they feel and behave in a particular way.

Clinical supervision can be viewed from the standpoint of such a traditional 'medical model', where the supervisee comes to supervision with problems. These problems are then solved by the supervisor. It is perhaps an attractive option for the supervisee, already used to a problem-orientated approach to nursing, for the supervisor, who can be in a position of authority and control, and for the organisation, which can feel secure that problems in practice are being attended to.

An alternative to the 'medical model' of psychotherapy is the solution-focused approach to therapy in clinical nursing practice (Hawkes et al 1993). Further examples can also be found in Chevalier (1995) and Saunders (1996). Solution-focused therapy is a method developed by De Shazer (1985) that concentrates on people's competence rather than their deficits, their strengths rather than their weaknesses, their possibilities rather than their limitations. This alternative approach to therapy could be adapted for an alternative model of clinical supervision that concentrates on the supervisee and the supervisor finding a description of a solution rather than attempting to analyse the supervisee's 'problem'.

Wilgosh et al (1994), citing Milton Erikson, sum up the potential of this approach for clinical supervision ('client' should be replaced by 'supervisee'): 'The client often knows what to do to solve his problem but does not know that he knows'.

This approach at the very least allows a method of questioning that enables supervisors and supervisees to think about solutions in a more proactive way, rather than focusing on why the problem has happened or is happening. It also supports Johns's (1996) premise that practitioners already have an idea of what good practice is, the contradiction between that and the way they practise forming the basis for reflective practice.

Compare how different Hayley's supervision earlier in the chapter would look when a proactive and solution-focused approach is applied to her practice story as opposed to a more traditional problem-orientated perspective. Some questions adapted from the first session of solution-focused therapy that could be used in clinical supervision are:

Suppose that, after we talk today, you go home and while you are asleep a miracle occurs and the problem that brought you here today disappears, is resolved, and because you are asleep you do not know that the miracle has happened.

- What would be the first sign in your clinical practice that would tell you that the miracle had occurred?
- Has there been a time recently that all or some of these things (the signs of the miracle) were happening?
- What were you doing differently then?

In what ways do you think the two approaches might affect Hayley's clinical practice?

What might be the implications for your own clinical supervision as a supervisee by adopting a more solution-focused approach?

A SKILLS-BASED CLINICAL SUPERVISOR SELF-ASSESSMENT TOOL

This chapter has covered a number of essential skills for the clinical supervisee, some of which you will already have in varying degrees as a practitioner. You may now wish to assess your own performance as a clinical supervisee, and a tool for doing so is given in the Appendix to this chapter. Reflecting on the tool with colleagues in supervision will help you become more consciously aware of how you use clinical supervision and whether you are using such limited time to the full. As one of the skills of being a supervisee is to be open to receive feedback on your clinical practice, you may wish to compare your self-assessment with your clinical supervisor to see if they also agree with you. Are there any major similarities or differences between the way you see yourself and the way your supervisor sees you?

On reflection ... chapter summary

What are the key elements of this chapter?

- Much of the clinical supervision literature concentrates on the development of the supervisor rather than that of the supervisee
- Supervisees, not supervisors, will determine the success, or lack of it, of clinical supervision in practice
- Supervisees must maximise their use of limited clinical supervision time
- Clinical supervision is metaphorically speaking an opportunity to share stories about clinical practice
- Clinical supervision is a way of helping the supervisee recognise his/her 'self' in clinical practice
- Writing regularly about things that happen in clinical practice can help the supervisee to choose issues to take to clinical supervision
- Clinical supervision is about finding solutions to the problems of clinical practice

So what difference does this make to the way I am operating my clinical/ supervisory practice?

Now what actions will need to be taken as a result of my reflections?

REFERENCES

Bishop V 1998 (ed) Clinical supervision in practice – some questions, answers and guidelines. Macmillan/Nursing Times Research, London

Bond M, Holland S 1998 Skills of clinical supervision for nurses. Open University Press, Buckingham

Bowles N 1995 Storytelling: a search for meaning within nursing practice. Nurse Education Today (15): 365–369

Butcher K 1995 Taking notes. Nursing Times 91(26): 33

Chevalier AJ 1995 On the clients path. A manual for the practice of solution focussed therapy. New Harbinger Publ, Oakland, California, USA

De Shazer S 1985 Keys to solutions in brief therapy. WW Norton, New York

Froggatt K 1998 The place of metaphor and language in exploring nurses' emotional work. Journal of Advanced Nursing 28(2): 332–338

Hawkes D, Wilgosh R, Marsh I 1993 Explaining solution focused therapy. Nursing Standard 7(33): 31–33

Heron J 1973 Experiential training techniques. Human Potential Research Project, University of Surrey, Guildford

Johns C 1996 Visualising and realising caring in practice through guided reflection. Journal of Advanced Nursing 24: 1135–1143

Johns C, Freshwater D (ed) 1998 Transforming nursing through reflective practice. Blackwell Science, Oxford

Marrow CE, Macauley DM, Crumbie A 1997 Promoting reflective practice through structured clinical supervision. Journal of Nursing Management (5): 77–82

McEvoy P 1993 A chance for feedback. Nursing Times 89(47): 55

Morrison P, Burnard P 1991 Caring and communicating: the interpersonal relationship in nursing. Macmillan, Basingstoke

New G, Cormack D 1997 Why did I do that? Understanding and mastering your motives. Hodder & Stoughton, London

Sams DA 1997 Clinical supervision: an evaluation of the implementation process within a community trust. BSc(Hons) dissertation, South Bank University, London

Saunders C 1996 Solution focused therapy in practice: a personal experience. Counselling (November): 312–316.

Seijo H 1996 Developing supervision in teams: a workbook for supervisors. Association of Practitioners in Learning Disabilities, Nottingham

Street A 1995 Nursing replay: researching nursing culture together. Churchill Livingstone, Edinburgh

UKCC 1996 Position statement on clinical supervision for nursing and health visiting. United Kingdom Central Council for Nursing, Midwifery and Health Visiting, London

UKCC 1997 PREP and you. United Kingdom Central Council for Nursing, Midwifery and Health Visiting, London

Vezeau T 1993 Storytelling: a practitioner's tool. American Journal of Maternal and Child Nursing 18: 193–196

Wilgosh R, Hawkes D, Marsh I 1994 Solution focused therapy in promoting mental health. Mental Health Nursing 14(6): 18–21

Appendix: Supervisee self-assessment tool

Read the following statements and tick the box that you feel most accurately reflects the statement in relation to your own supervisory practice.

Questionnaire

Statement		Always	Sometimes	Never
1.	I let the supervisor open the session	❏	❏	❏
2.	I let the supervisor know what the session will be about	❏	❏	❏
3.	I spend time thinking about the session beforehand	❏	❏	❏
4.	I ask the supervisor to alter aspects of the session I am unhappy about	❏	❏	❏
5.	I leave the supervision session more able to deal with practice concerns	❏	❏	❏
6.	I can work out what practice stories to recount in the supervision session	❏	❏	❏
7.	I make a note of different things that happen in practice that will be useful in supervision	❏	❏	❏
8.	Part of the session usually involves time to clarify the documentation	❏	❏	❏
9.	I talk to the supervisor about things that went well in my practice	❏	❏	❏
10.	I talk about my supervison concerns to others prior to the session	❏	❏	❏
11.	The supervisor can make me feel uncomfortable about what I do in my clinical practice	❏	❏	❏
12.	Supervision sessions help me focus on my feelings about clinical practice	❏	❏	❏
13.	I am a thoughtful clinical practitioner in supervision	❏	❏	❏
14.	I am a thoughtful practitioner in my clinical practice	❏	❏	❏
15.	I see how what is discussed in clinical supervision relates to me as a practitioner	❏	❏	❏
16.	I view clinical supervision as a positive learning experience	❏	❏	❏
17.	I act on what I hear during the session from the clinical supervisor	❏	❏	❏
18.	I am not offended by the feedback my supervisor gives me	❏	❏	❏
19.	I thank the supervisor for being open with me at the end of the session	❏	❏	❏
20.	I ask the supervisor for feedback on specific elements of my clinical practice	❏	❏	❏
21.	I write about my clinical practice other than the usual nursing documentation at the end of a shift	❏	❏	❏
22.	I write up my clinical supervision sessions and keep a record of them	❏	❏	❏
23.	I prepare for the session ahead by writing down what I wish to talk about	❏	❏	❏
24.	I store my clinical supervision notes in my professional portfolio	❏	❏	❏

Questionnaire (Cont.)

Statement	Always	Sometimes	Never
25. I use a reflective framework when writing up my supervision notes	❏	❏	❏
26. I talk about my problems regarding clinical practice in the supervision session	❏	❏	❏
27. I talk about problems regarding clinical practice in the supervision session that really belong to others	❏	❏	❏
28. Clinical supervision concentrates on my competence and strengths as a practitioner	❏	❏	❏
29. I have an idea of how I would like my clinical practice to look and discuss this in the supervision sessions	❏	❏	❏
30. My clinical supervision focuses on solutions rather than problems	❏	❏	❏

Score each answer on the answer grid below. Give yourself 3 marks for Always, 2 marks for Sometimes and 1 mark for Never. Total the scores for each baseline skill. The maximum score for each of the six skills is 15, the minimum score is 5. Enter the total scores from each question into the table and see how you have done.

Answer grid

Baseline skills of the supervisee	Ability to make the session work for you	Ability to identify pertinent stories to disclose	Awareness of your 'self' in clinical practice	Willingness to receive feedback	Ability to write as well as talk about practice	Ability to be proactive in seeking practice solutions
Question no. Your score	2	6	3	1	7	5
Question no. Your score	4	9	12	11	8	10
Question no. Your score	14	15	13	17	21	20
Question no. Your score	28	25	16	18	22	23
Question no. Your score	29	26	27	19	24	30
Maximum score	15	15	15	15	15	15
Your total score						
Minimum score	5	5	5	5	5	5

You have now formed your personal baseline from which to begin to think about gauging your performance as a clinical supervisee. On reflection, what sort of things have you learned and need to action in your clinical supervision?

You may wish to do this exercise again in 6 months' time to chart your progress as a clinical supervisee.

© Harcourt Publishers Limited 2000

7 Essential skills for clinical supervisors

INTRODUCTION

Much of this book has been about different hopes, fears and expectations of clinical supervision in the context of practice. It is relatively easy to theorise about what occurs during the clinical supervision encounter and to produce endless lists of roles, responsibilities and potential benefits and burdens, but what is it that needs to happen? The danger in worrying about whether you are doing it 'right' or whether it aligns with some theory or other is that clinical supervision becomes so complicated that it can put individuals off doing it at all!

Clinical supervision is essentially an activity in which the supervisor already has some skills in the 'doing' of everyday nursing practice that can readily be transferred to the clinical supervision encounter. The trick is in actively noticing what you already do as a practitioner that might form the essential skills of a clinical supervisor. The unquestioning borrowing of counselling, psychotherapy, midwifery and social work supervisory knowledge, while initially helpful, must not limit the development of more specific knowledge of supervision as it relates to nursing and health visiting.

This chapter is by no means an exhaustive list of the skills of a clinical supervisor, but is put forward as a summary of some of the essential skills required. These are gleaned from my own experiences as a clinical supervisor, and supervising clinical supervisors, and of those of course participants in clinical supervisor training workshops and the ENB RO1 course (Clinical Supervision Skills for Clinical Supervisors).

For certain specialisms in nursing, e.g. mental health and learning disabilities, a more psychotherapeutic approach to supervision is required; this is already developing and is beyond the scope of this book, although an overview of different supervisory styles and approaches is given in a later chapter. The essential skills outlined may therefore be a re-formulation of what nurses already do, but a genuine invitation is also extended to collaborate with adult nursing colleagues in the development of their supervisory knowledge and skills.

THE ANATOMY OF A CLINICAL SUPERVISION SESSION

In previous chapters a basic structure for organising clinical supervision sessions was put forward. This forms a useful framework for starting to identify the essential skills of the clinical supervisor. It may be helpful to remind yourself of the anatomy of an ongoing clinical supervision session (Box 7.1), as opposed to the initial contractual concerns of the first session. You may wish to add other points that seem important to you from your supervisor workshops.

BOX 7.1	*The anatomy of a clinical supervision session from a clinical supervisor's point of view*

Adequately prepare before the supervisee arrives

- Prepare for session by reminding oneself what went on previously
- Ensure a conducive environment
- Start the session on time
- Other points you may wish to add?

After the supervisee has arrived and is settled

- Review what went on in the previous session and follow up issues where necessary
- Find out how each other is feeling before agreeing on a fresh agenda
- Prioritise the agenda for the session
- Other points you may wish to add?

During the session

- Allow supervisee to describe the issue(s) to the supervisor
- Supervisor listens and gives feedback to the supervisee
- Jointly analyse issues and work out together ways of moving forward
- Other points you may wish to add?

Towards the end of the session

- Supervisor clarifies and summarises what has been discussed in the session
- Record session as previously agreed
- Ask supervisee for feedback on supervisor performance
- Check date/time/venue for next session

Close the session

IDENTIFYING SKILLS TRANSFERABLE FROM CLINICAL PRACTICE THAT COULD BE USED BY A CLINICAL SUPERVISOR

It is probably evident from Box 7.1 that as a practitioner you already have some experience of guiding a supervision session of sorts, e.g. formatively assessing preregistration students, handling complaints, having a discussion with a relative about a patient/client diagnosis, or reviewing a patient/client in a formal setting such as a case conference or ward round.

How does some of what you already do in practice equate to the skills of a clinical supervisor? How transferable could they be into the clinical supervision situation?

You may wish to compare some of your own ideas to my list in Box 7.2, which is based on the anatomy of a clinical supervision session.

The number of transferable skills might have surprised you. Many of them you may not have even noticed, or did not regard as particularly special. Helping supervisees notice the unnoticed (Street 1995) in clinical practice is a specific remit of the clinical supervisor. Noticing your own skills potentially transferable to clinical supervision will help you to adapt, rather than just adopt, clinical supervision into your work area.

SIX ESSENTIAL SKILLS OF A CLINICAL SUPERVISOR

Although much of the literature purports to tell you what clinical supervision skills are, you should always consider them in relation to what you are doing already. There is no agreed way of doing clinical supervision in nursing in general, particularly not in the area in which you work. Even if you are fortunate enough to have managerial backing to undertake clinical supervision in your practice area, what actually goes on will depend on the skills of the supervisee as well as the supervisor. It is therefore important to first identify things that go well in supervision, develop these skills and disseminate them to others. In this way a body of supervision knowledge will begin to emerge in nursing that is based on critically reflecting on the process of supervision.

On the basis of some early work in workshops with supervisees and supervisors, six essential skills are identified (Box 7.3) for giving effective supervision.

It is unlikely that every supervisor will be competent in each of these at first, but they are likely to be considered in initial clinical supervisor training. These can then be added to, if the supervisor wishes, through further reading or more advanced courses in supervision. Much will depend on the supervisory style or approach adopted.

BOX 7.2	*Some transferable supervisory skills from clinical practice*
Anatomy of a supervision session (from Box .7.1)	**Transferable practice skills that can be used by the supervisor**
Adequately preparing for practice storytelling beforehand	**Record keeping** **Care planning** **Personal time management** **Liaising with colleagues**
Prepare for session by reminding oneself what went on previously	**Organisational**, e.g. filing session notes, record keeping **Memory**, e.g. remembering the person in supervision
Supervisor has a responsibility for ensuring a conducive environment	**Managerial**, e.g. checking venue – too hot, cold, noisy – coffee? **Interruption control/privacy**, e.g. do not disturb sign, pager/phone off or diverted, door closed, out of earshot of others
Start the session on time	**Time management**, e.g. session planned, anticipated, demonstration of a **commitment to clinical supervision** in busy work schedule
Review what went on in the previous session and follow up issues where necessary	**Relationship skills**, e.g. giving full attention, **re-establishing the supervision partnership, clarifying** what went on before
Find out how the other is feeling before agreeing on a fresh agenda	**Self-awareness**, e.g. obstacles to effective communication and reflective practice, genuineness
Prioritise the agenda	**Understanding** of the function of clinical supervision
Supervisee describes the issue(s) to the supervisor	**Relationship skills**, e.g. acceptance, being **non-judgemental, facilitation of reflective practice**
Supervisor listens and gives feedback to the supervisee	**Active listening skills**, e.g. understanding how to give **effective feedback** to the supervisee
Jointly analyse issues and work out together ways of moving forward	**Analytical skills**, e.g. **questioning** technique, **intervention style**
Supervisor clarifies and summarises what has been discussed in the session	**Understanding how the supervisee can learn** from the experience of clinical supervision **Summarising skills** **Active listening** during the session **Intervention style**

| BOX 7.2 (Cont.) | Some transferable supervisory skills from clinical practice |

Anatomy of a supervision session (from Box .7.1)	Transferable practice skills that can be used by the supervisor
Record session as previously agreed	**Relationship skills**, e.g. trust, **Confidentiality**, honouring or revisiting agreements made in the first session as regards documentation and recording
Ask supervisee for feedback on supervisor performance	**Accepting feedback**, e.g. being open, non-defensive and **willing to learn** from the supervisee **Being aware of how supervisor performance can be evaluated**
Check date/time/venue for next session	**Organisational skills Intervention style Commitment** to supervisory role

| BOX 7.3 | Six essential skills for clinical supervisors |

- Open an emotional supervisory account
- Be willing to mutually learn from engaging in clinical supervision
- Be attentive to what is going on in the session
- Use effective questioning to help supervisees notice themselves in clinical practice
- Be open to receive as well as give feedback on practice
- Be able to summarise the content of the session with the supervisee

Essential skill 1: Open an emotional supervisory account

All relationships progress through phases regardless of whether the relationship is with a person, a project or a setting. Intuitively, it is probably apparent that therapeutic relationships in clinical practice, as well as personal relationships, flourish or flounder according to whether both parties perceive themselves as becoming connected or 'disconnected' in some way.

In supervision, the supervisee and supervisor take on roles and tasks that are required for the relationship to progress or flounder. Covey (1992) uses the metaphor of an emotional bank account to describe the development of relationships, and this is a useful way of considering the supervision relationship:

In a financial bank account we make deposits into it and build up a reserve from which we can make withdrawals when we need to. An emotional bank account describes the amount of trust that has been built up in a relationship. Its the feeling of safeness you have with another human being. Deposits such as courtesy, kindness, honesty and being committed build up a reserve. Your trust towards me becomes higher and I can call upon that trust many times if I need to. When the trust account is high communication is easy, instant and effective. If I have a habit of showing discourtesy, disrespect, cutting you off, betraying your trust eventually my emotional bank account gets very low. To be sustained continuing deposits are necessary (Covey 1992, p. 188).

Continuing the bank account metaphor, some personal reflections may help you notice why, as a supervisor, making emotional deposits in the supervisory relationship is an essential baseline skill for an effective supervision partnership.

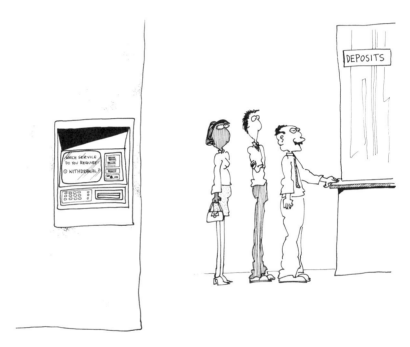

History Box   I find the easiest type of transaction is to pull up on a double yellow line and quickly **withdraw** from the hole-in-the-wall before I can be accosted by a traffic warden. I can get away with being overdrawn a little bit and do not have to face the bank teller in any event! There is also a sense of satisfaction in having got away with illegal parking when others are looking for a space in the multistorey or had to put money in a parking meter!

Making **deposits** in my bank account (which I don't do that often), requires a conscious effort on my part. I do not feel safe placing money in a hole in the wall in case the computer messes up and I lose my money, so I have to physically go to the bank. Usually this visit occurs after a threatening letter from the bank, or when I want to change some sterling for a foreign holiday. Although this way is safer, I have to make the effort to find time in working hours, make pleasant conversation when I often do not wish to and have my finances scrutinised by the bank teller, who I hope will not let the rest of the queue behind me know of my poor financial management. Sometimes this may end with a rather guilty apology on my part.

Think of a patient/person you are involved with in practice that, as a practitioner, you find challenging. What would your emotional bank statement look like as regards deposits and withdrawals if you asked that patient/person to make up your account as a nurse? Write down the 'deposits' and 'withdrawals' in two columns.

Conversely, think of a patient/person you are involved with in practice whom you really like. What would your emotional bank statement look like as regards deposits and withdrawals if you asked that patient/person to make up your account as a nurse?

You might like to compare your thoughts with some deposits and withdrawals a supervisor might make in the clinical supervision bank account during a session (Box 7.4).

What might be the implications of these for the clinical supervisor?

BOX 7.4	*The clinical supervision bank statement*

Some supervisory deposits:

- Being committed to the supervisee
  'If I could come over to your area for the supervision session, rather than you coming over to me, it would help me greatly in understanding your clinical situation.'
- Noticing the supervisee
  'Would a change in the session time help you to wind down before supervision?… I've made you a coffee.'
- Gaining an understanding of how the supervisee feels
  'Although you are laughing at the situation now, I suspect that the situation really upset you at the time.'
- Showing personal integrity
  'I'm not going to talk about [the person you refer to] behind their back. I'm sure you would not wish me to do that about something you said.'
- Apologising unreservedly after having made a mistake
  'I'm sorry that you felt that I embarrassed you in the last session…. My intention was to challenge you, not embarrass you. Thank you feeling able to tell me…. I'll need to think about how I conduct supervision sessions in the future…. How do you think we can avoid this?'

Some supervisory withdrawals:

- Cutting off the supervisee's experience in favour of what you think should happen
  'The same happened to me once, and I think you should…'
- Blaming and penalising without concern for the supervisee
  'I'll have to hurry up this session because you're late and I've got an important meeting this afternoon.'
- Concentrating on other things and obvious lack of interest in the supervisee
  'Sorry, can you hang on a minute? I need to speak to Dr X as she's in the clinic…. I'm off home after this session and I'll miss her.'
- Failure to keep confidentiality and demonstrating a lack of trust towards the supervisee
  'It's a bit embarrassing that you found out I had spoken to the link tutor about that course you enquired about in the last session…. He never comes to the ward normally.'

Essential skill 2: Be willing to mutually learn from engaging in clinical supervision

Previous chapters examined how the principles of adult learning in the formalised process of clinical supervision offer the supervisor, as well as the supervisee, an opportunity to review and rediscover clinical practice. An enquiring approach to everyday practice, whether in clinical practice as a supervisee or in supervisory practice as a supervisor, is a fundamental skill for achieving effective clinical supervision.

Although this skill might be regarded as obvious and one that everybody in nursing acquires anyway, is this really the case? I would suggest that it is by no means straightforward in nursing cultures where people are often 'too busy' to talk to patients and clients in any meaningful way, and sometimes even to one another.

In traditional models of learning, a hierarchy exists in which those who supposedly have knowledge transmit it to a willing learner who does not. In clinical supervision I would argue that the supervisor must be willing to learn from the supervisee. Nursing is still a long way from developing specific supervision knowledge and therefore a specific supervisory skill is to be willing to learn from the supervisee, resisting the temptation to be 'in charge' of supervision knowledge.

In a busy professional life that places demands on the qualified practitioner to be accountable as well as clinically effective, being reflective might seem to be a luxury. I would suggest that some form of systematic reflection like clinical supervision may be the only opportunity nurses have to professionally develop. Without some way of reviewing practice not only are practitioners disadvantaged but so are the patients being looked after.

A useful framework for understanding how the supervisor can learn as well as the supervisee is to consider whether you demonstrate a need for learning (the incompetence element) and are aware of the need to learn (the consciousness factor). O'Connor & Seymour (1993, p. 8) describe four different stages of learning based on whether you consider yourself to be competent or not and whether you are actually aware of the need to learn. If you are a new clinical supervisor you may wish to consider which of the four quadrants shown in Figure 7.1 you are currently in.

Presumably if you are already a clinical supervisor reading this book, you are conscious of the need to learn more and feel incompetent (or that you should become more competent) about clinical supervision. You will therefore be in the two quadrants most ripe for learning – consciously incompetent or consciously competent. As a clinical supervisor it is useful to aim to achieve a state of 'conscious incompetence' in a supervisee during a session. In this learning state the supervisee will be or become aware of the need to learn further about a particular aspect of their practice.

Read the following four statements which might have been made in a clinical supervision session. If one of your essential skills is to help the supervisee learn, into which learning quadrant of Figure 7.2 would you class the maker of each statement and, more importantly, what might be the implications for you as a clinical supervisor if you were conducting the session?

| Figure 7.1 | *Four different stages of learning* |

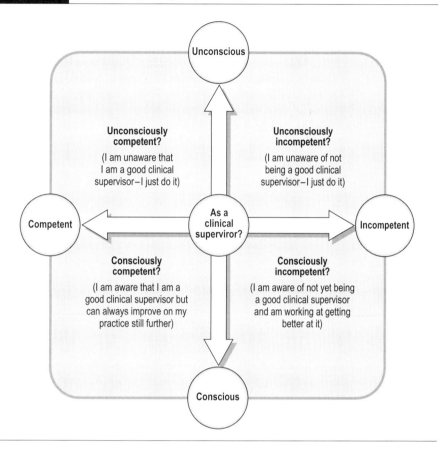

'I couldn't understand it – the night nurse manager went mad at me when I said I had switched off the alarm on Mr Jones's infusion pump because it kept going off and disturbing all the patients.... At least all my patients then managed to have a good night's sleep and I could get the paperwork done for the early shift!'

'I started to feel really stupid – one or two of the patients were continually shouting out that they couldn't get to sleep because of the bleeping of the infusion pump.... I played around with it for a bit to try to get it to work properly ... after a few minutes I worried that the analgesia might not be working, although Mr Jones said he wasn't in any pain.... In the end I switched it off and phoned the senior staff nurse on the other ward to come over and show me what to do.... The battery was low and we changed over to a mains lead.'

'I met the senior staff nurse at breakfast in the canteen and apologised for calling her over to the ward – she had been having a hellish night with so many admissions.... She told me where the operator's handbook was in the office, so I asked the charge nurse if she could get the ward clerk to photocopy the pages dealing with alarms and troubleshooting problems for me ... and perhaps as Jenny, my senior staff nurse, is back from leave tomorrow tonight she'll go through the pump with me after I've had a chance to read up a bit more about it.'

'I was really cheesed off ... we were having a hellish night when I got called out to sort out an infusion pump that kept on going off across the way.... Luckily, it only took a second.... This Trust is really sailing close to the wind when we leave a junior staff nurse in charge of such an acute ward.... Anyway, I've been asked to set up this induction package for new staff.'

Figure 7.2	*Four different stages of learning for the supervisee*

As the examples illustrate, supervisees come to the session with different levels of awareness and competence. If the supervisee is willing to learn and become more aware of their deficiencies, it is relatively straightforward to manoeuvre them into situations and ways of further learning. This is how clinical supervision can enhance clinical practice, through formalised and critical reflection on clinical practice.

A management agenda for clinical supervision that is not unreasonable, given the support for it in practice, is for the clinical supervisor to be alert to assessing the clinical risk that members of staff may represent for their patients (Naish 1995, Tingle 1995). The risk for healthcare organisations of litigation and poor publicity will, it is envisaged, be reduced by the supervisor helping supervisees become more consciously aware of what they do, as well as what they do not seem to do. In this way, clinical supervision could also be said to be a vehicle for clinical governance by ensuring that nursing work is of a high quality (Department of Health 1998). By willingly engaging in clinical supervision, both the supervisor and the supervisee are actually demonstrating clinical governance in practice.

Being attentive to what goes on in the supervision session is particularly important for a supervisor when dealing with staff who seem blissfully ignorant of the consequences of incompetent practice. Often this is unconscious and can occur in staff members who appear to be already competent. How many seem to miss out on in-house updates or are 'too busy' or 'too senior' to further their learning or professional development?

Essential skill 3: Be attentive to what is going on in the session

Purely by virtue of being human, the clinical supervisor has a number of abilities at his/her disposal to find out what makes the supervisee tick in clinical practice, and most do it without really thinking about it. That's the problem – we take too much for granted! As O'Connor & Seymour (1993, p. 3) put it: 'We organise what we hear, feel and see by editing and filtering the outside world through our senses (sight, hearing, touch, smell and taste) ... everyone lives in their own unique reality built from their sense impressions and individual experiences of life, and we *act on the basis of what we perceive our model of the world to be.*'

Despite having a range of life and individual experience and five sensory pathways, some safe assumptions can be made about you as a supervisor, and these constitute some of the pitfalls of the role:

■ You will often not be conscious of intentionally using your senses in the clinical supervision session

■ You will tend to view the supervisee according to your own model of the situation the supervisee is describing, rather than as the supervisee is describing it

■ You are very likely to rush in with quick-fix solutions for the supervisee before listening and understanding what the situation really is.

One way of demonstrating in supervision that you are attentive to what is going on is to listen properly. You can make sure that you are doing this (or not) by checking with the supervisee, preferably during the session. Covey (1992, pp. 236–259) suggests that most people do not listen with the intent to understand, they listen with the intent to reply: 'They are either speaking or preparing to reply. They are filtering everything through their own home movies onto other people's behaviour.... "Oh, I know exactly how you feel" ... in other words prescribing what they see to whom they interact with before making a diagnosis of what is really going on.'

One can imagine a surgeon, optician, dentist or general practitioner being struck off the register for prescribing something to a patient without first fully diagnosing the medical condition. They are at more risk if, in doing so, they give the wrong treatment and in further trouble if this leads to a formal complaint or litigation.

In clinical supervision, but also in any meaningful communication in clinical practice, actively listening will help you to make a positive diagnosis (metaphorically speaking) before a prescription is given. As Burnard (1996, p. 74) says, we rarely need a definition of listening as we have all experienced it and know what it is. In clinical supervision, the supervisor, through actively listening, is not only showing an interest in the supervisee but is more likely to more accurately recall what was spoken about.

Active listening differs from ordinary listening in a number of different ways. Briefly describe the behaviours you as a supervisor can use to demonstrate to the supervisee that you are actively listening, as opposed to ordinary listening. How do these compare to my list in Box 7.5?

BOX 7.5	Differences in supervisor behaviour when actively listening to the supervisee rather than ordinary listening

Active listening	Ordinary listening
Conscious effort made	Unconscious effort made
Paying little attention to how what you hear relates to yourself	Relating what you hear to yourself
Attention to what is not being said	Attention to what is intended to be heard
Interest in verbal and non-verbal communication	Interest in verbal communication
Unhurried approach to listening	Constantly interrupting flow
Body language demonstrates interest	Listening while doing something else
Maintaining acceptable eye contact	Easily distracted by external factors
Encouraging interventions, e.g. 'Yes, go on'	Needing to be reminded of what has been said

Active listening means that a conscious effort is made not only to listen to the words employed by the supervisee but also to pick up non-verbal cues indicating the speaker's reaction to the situation being spoken about. Your own listening behaviours as a supervisor can also be picked up by the supervisee while they are talking and enhance, or limit, the conversation.

Imagine what a supervisee would feel like if, having had difficulty in arranging clinical supervision, they arrive, prepared, to be confronted by a supervisor who appears uninterested or preoccupied with something else. It is very unlikely that the supervisee would wish to waste precious time with you again – quite apart from what they might tell others about your supervisory technique! Such behaviour would undoubtedly constitute a withdrawal from the supervision bank account.

Essential skill 4: Use effective questioning to help the supervisee notice 'him/herself' in clinical practice

Questioning by the supervisor in clinical supervision can both reveal and limit the work of the clinical practitioner. A starting point for asking questions in clinical supervision could be to consider just what it is you are setting out to do by having what might be considered to be a professional conversation with a practitioner about their practice. If the aim of clinical supervision is not clear for either the supervisor or the supervisee then the responses to questions set by the supervisor can be misinterpreted or become guarded.

Ewles & Simnett (1999, p. 188) distinguish between four common types of question:

- **Closed questions,** which require short, factual, often one-word answers
- **Open questions,** which offer more opportunity for fuller answers
- **Biased questions,** which indicate the preferable response
- **Multiple questions,** which contain more than one question.

Closed questions can be appropriate in supervision:

'Is the room too cold?'

'Did you bring your documentation from the last session?'

'Can I borrow your pen – mine has run out?'

However, they are not appropriate if the supervisor is trying to encourage the supervisee to talk about specific aspects of clinical practice in more detail. Sometimes supervisees are grateful that the question the supervisor puts to them only requires a one-word answer, as they may not wish to elaborate:

Supervisor: 'Did you manage to speak to the tutor about the course you were interested in?'

Supervisee: 'No, not yet.'

Another way of expressing the same question might be to use a question of a more open type. Open questions are generally more appropriate in supervision as they allow for fuller answers and more elaboration:

Supervisor: 'How did you find the course tutor you said you were going to speak to about that course?'

Supervisee: 'Well, to be honest, I've been so busy in the clinic that it completely slipped my mind until yesterday.'

This can then invite another follow-up question by the supervisor:

'What do you feel about doing a course when you are so busy in the clinic at the moment?'

A biased or leading question might have been a bad alternative to the follow-up question. In this, the supervisor indicates within the question the answer she/he expects – but there is usually a get-out clause for the supervisee:

Supervisor: 'You didn't forget to speak to the course tutor as you said you would, did you?'

Supervisee: 'It's in hand.'

The supervisor now has to consider whether it is worth being confrontational by asking more probing questions to clarify the situation, or whether the matter is not important enough to pursue, since it has been raised again with the supervisee.

A multiple question might be tempting, as it offers to possibility of clarifying everything at once, but is only likely to appeal to the supervisor while confusing or angering the supervisee:

Supervisor: 'How do you think not speaking to the tutor about getting on the Teaching and Assessing course will affect your promotion chances – you brought the issue up last time because you wanted to improve your teaching practice with junior students and a senior staff nurse post was imminent?'

Supervisee: I'm not quite sure what you're getting at ... look, I forgot to speak to her, OK. Is that a crime?'

Questions are a useful tool for the clinical supervisor but you need to be clear as to why and for what purpose the question is being asked in the first place. Most questions in clinical supervision will be to:

- Encourage the supervisee to open up about specific aspects of their practice:
  'Can you tell me a bit more about how you, rather than the ward team, felt about what happened?'

- Clarify issues:
  'I'm sorry, did you say you were going to meet the patient's relatives again?'

- Get some more information about the situation described:
  'What made you so angry with the doctor?'

- Explore a situation with the supervisee in more depth:
  'I'm sure that the whole incident must have upset you at the time – in what ways do you think that it has had a bearing on your practice since then?'

Questions are also a useful way of checking levels of actual or potential learning (see above). The responses to questions posed in a conversational rather than an inquisitorial way also form the basis of clear and effective feedback to the supervisee on elements of their clinical practice. This is one of the responsibilities of the clinical supervisor (Chapter 5).

In order for feedback to be effective you, the supervisor, need to ensure that you have obtained a clear understanding of what was discussed and are not simply viewing the situation according to your own perception of what probably happened. Questioning is therefore a useful aid to more fully validate the supervisor's understanding of the supervisee's situation.

Essential skill 5: Be open to receive as well as give feedback on practice

One of the functions of clinical supervision is to maintain and enhance standards and the quality of the nursing delivered by the practitioner (UKCC 1996). The vehicle for doing so is effective feedback given to the supervisee by the supervisor. McEvoy (1993) notes that, before clinical supervision was introduced, many nurses on the unit studied felt that they were only told when their clinical performance was not up to scratch and were given little positive feedback.

As Seijo (1996, p. 50) rightly points out, it is not sufficient simply to give staff feedback on performance that could be improved, it is also essential to highlight what is being performed well, in order to maintain morale and reinforce that behaviour. In other words, giving and receiving feedback on performance can be positive as well as negative.

As clinical supervision in practice is still in its infancy, it is fair to say that clinical supervisors also must be open to critical comment from the supervisee on their performance. It might be interesting to tape or video a session to compare the similarities between giving and receiving feedback from the supervisor to the supervisee and from the supervisee to the supervisor. This is a central part of any clinical supervisor training workshop, although the course participants are often embarrassed and surprised at first by watching and getting feedback on performance. In the real situation, of course, the supervisor has the primary responsibility for giving feedback.

When was the last time you received any feedback on the work you do?
  What do you remember most about it?
  Who gave it and why?
  When was the last time you *asked* for some specific feedback on the work you do?
  What do you remember most about it?
  Who gave it and why?
  Were there any similarities or differences between the two types of feedback? How does your idea of not-so-good feedback compare with the examples of feedback to a supervisee given in Box 7.6?

Good practice points in giving effective feedback

Like all the other baseline skills, giving feedback requires some practice, perhaps even some feedback on how you did it, or how it made the other person feel at the time. Clinical supervision feedback is different from the type of feedback you often give as a manager or when you are assessing a student nurse's competencies in order to pass a placement. Dolley et al (1998) suggest that constructive feedback is best given like a sandwich, with the negative in between two slices of positive!

BOX 7.6	*What clinical supervisory feedback is not*

- A punitive or disciplinary procedure
- Insinuating that the supervisee practitioner is a failure
- Criticism for the sake of it – 'I have to find something wrong'
- Manipulating the supervisee into acting as you think they should
- Confusing to the supervisee
- A way of maintaining authority in the supervisory relationship
- An inaccurate account of what has gone on
- A blaming exercise to get the supervisee to change their practice

It is likely that:

- the supervisee will be expecting some feedback from you
- it is part of your supervisory role to give it
- persistently negative feedback will put the supervisee off returning to you again and you'll gain a reputation in supervisee circles!
- clinical supervision is a professional conversation (Jones 1998), not an assessment of an already qualified practitioner.

Supervisee workshops, as well as supervisor workshops, are now inviting participants to consider not only how to receive but also how to give feedback (Tate 1998). Such workshops are a useful opportunity to explore how to give feedback, identify clearly what we want to say, be clear about our motives and practise the skills for verbalising it, as well as, importantly, learning to deal with different reactions to it.

Feedback is not failure. Failure is another way of describing something you did not anticipate or want to happen. Feedback is an opportunity to learn from something you had not noticed, but somebody else did.

Here are some more effective examples of feedback statements, based on the work of Seijo (1996, p. 51):

- Be responsible as a supervisor for the supervisee by personally owning, rather than generalising, the feedback given:
  'I imagine that you would have preferred not to have spoken to the doctor in that way, but I think I can understand why you did.'
- The feedback statement needs to refer to observed, rather than assumed behaviours:
  'I noticed that you slammed the door when you came into the room just now – is it right to say you are angry about something that happened recently?'
- Be specific about the behaviour you are giving feedback about, rather than just saying that something was 'good':
  'You seemed unconvinced when you said that the charge nurse was pleased with your management of that difficult staff member – in fact you raised your eyebrows and gave a little sigh as you were telling me.'

- The behaviour referred to needs to be something that the supervisee is able to adapt or change, rather than something where change is not feasible:
'I have become aware that you are persistently arriving late for the supervision session – for the last two sessions over 15 minutes late. What could you do to improve your timing, as the session is now only 45 minutes long instead of the hour we originally agreed?'

- Give feedback as soon as possible after it has been heard or observed in the session:
'I noticed that you are a bit unsure of what you have just said – why might that be?'

- Encourage the supervisee to be specific about what aspect of the situation described they want feedback on:
'In what way can I help you with the situation you have just described to me?'

- Aim to give the supervisee an element of choice during the feedback: the more choices or options open to the supervisee the better the exploration of the situation:
'From what we have discussed there appear to be two main options open to you – have you also thought about it from the point of view of how the patient might be feeling?'

- Ask for the supervisee to give you feedback on both your performance in giving feedback and your behaviour with them in supervision:
'It would be really helpful for my own supervision if you could make me aware of how I have performed as a clinical supervisor today.'

Essential skill 6: Be able to summarise the content of the session with the supervisee

Johns (1996) in his definition of reflection, always points the 'reflector' (in this case the supervisee) towards seeing the contradictions between desirable clinical practice and the way that s/he actually does practise. The identified contradictions can form the basis for a useful discussion in clinical supervision. Part of the skill of the supervisor is then to be able to summarise for the supervisee what has gone on in the session. An obvious conflict in supervisory practice arises when you try to recall accurately what the supervisee has said while also trying to concentrate on the whole of what is going on in the session!

Some supervisors negotiate with the supervisee a way of doing this by using audiovisual aids, or simply a paper and a pencil in the early stages. Always try to validate your own summary of what has gone on in the session with the supervisee. Summarising the session is not dissimilar to writing a concluding chapter or the final couple of paragraphs of a report. Neither require an over-complex replay of the whole experience, just to touch on the main learning points that have been raised. If the supervisor has been giving feedback continually throughout the session, it is not necessary to cover all the points in detail again.

Butterworth et al (1997, pp. 29–35), in a substantial study, offer a tentative list of issues important enough to be raised in clinical supervision sessions (Box 7.7).

BOX 7.7	*Issues raised in supervision sessions that might form the basis of the supervisor's summary*

- Clinical casework
- Organisational and management issues
- Confidence building
- Professional development
- Educational support
- Personal matters
- Interpersonal problems

While this is a useful aide-memoire for new supervisors, it is unlikely to cover all the complex issues that can be raised in supervision sessions. However, the list might be useful as major headings to summarise from.

The key point to remember in summarising the session is to be alert to what is being said and the supervisee's reaction to it. It is of particular importance to check it with the supervisee for accuracy. Included in the summary will be what the supervisee intends to do to change the aspect(s) of clinical practice that they felt was important enough to bring to the session.

A SKILLS-BASED CLINICAL SUPERVISOR SELF-ASSESSMENT TOOL

This chapter has covered a number of essential skills for the clinical supervisor, which some of you will already have in varying degrees from working as a practitioner. You may now wish to assess your own performance as a clinical supervisor, and a tool for doing this is given in the Appendix to this chapter. While this exercise might be interesting in itself, it could also form the basis for feedback in your own supervision. Reflecting on the tool with others will help you become more consciously aware of your own performance as a supervisor and highlight areas to develop. If you are open enough to give feedback you may wish to compare your own assessment with your supervisees' assessment of you or in conjunction with any audiovisual aids you use in supervision. Are there any major similarities or differences?

This chapter has suggested to the clinical supervisor six essential skills required in giving effective clinical supervision – you are likely to discover more. Perhaps it has also formed a baseline from which to begin to think about gauging your own performance in supervision. On reflection, what sort of things have you learned about clinical supervision from a supervisor's perspective?

On reflection ... chapter summary

What are the key elements of this chapter?

- Theorising about the right way to do clinical supervision can put supervisors and supervisees off starting it at all

- Both clinical supervisors and supervisees already have some skills that they bring to supervision from clinical practice

- Noticing skills that can be transferred from practice to clinical supervision will help practitioners adapt rather than adopt supervisory strategies into nursing practice

- There is as yet no agreed way of doing clinical supervision in practice, only guiding principles

- Successful clinical supervision is dependent on the relationship that exists between the supervisor and supervisee

- Clinical supervision is a shared learning opportunity

- Clinical supervision is an opportunity to get feedback on clinical practice and is one of the roles of the clinical supervisor

So what difference does this make to the way I am operating my clinical/ supervisory practice?

Now what actions will need to be taken as a result of my reflections?

REFERENCES

Burnard P 1996 Acquiring interpersonal skills: a handbook of experiential learning for health professionals, 2nd edn. Chapman & Hall, London

Butterworth T, Carson J, White E, Jeacock A, Clements A, Bishop V 1997 It is good to talk. An evaluation study in England and Scotland. School of Nursing, Midwifery and Health Visiting, University of Manchester, Manchester

Covey SR 1992 The seven habits of highly effective people. Simon & Schuster, London

Department of Health 1998 A first class service – quality in the new NHS. 13175 NUR 13k 1P (June). Stationery Office, London

Dolley J, Davies C, Murray P 1998 Clinical supervision: a development pack for nurses (K509). Open University Press, Buckingham

Ewles L, Simnett I 1999 Promoting health – a practical guide, 4th edn. Baillière Tindall, in association with the Royal College of Nursing, London

Johns C 1996 Visualising and realising caring in practice through guided reflection. Journal of Advanced Nursing 24: 1135–1143

Jones A 1998 Building professional relationships. Nursing Times learning curve 2(4): 12–13

McEvoy P 1993 A chance for feedback. Nursing Times 89(47): 55

Naish J 1995 Clinical supervision – can you trust nurses' professional MOTs? Health Care Risk Report July/August: 16–17

O'Connor J, Seymour J 1993 Introducing NLP – neuro linguistic programming, revised edn. Aquarian Press, London

Seijo H 1996 Developing supervision in teams. A workbook for supervisors. Association of Practitioners in Learning Disabilities, Nottingham

Street A 1995 Nursing replay: researching nursing culture together. Churchill Livingstone, Edinburgh

Tate S 1998 Helping supervisees to get the most out of their supervisory experience. Nursing Times Learning Curve 2(2): 10–11

Tingle J 1995 Clinical supervision is an effective risk management tool. British Journal of Nursing 4(14): 794–795

UKCC 1996 Position statement on clinical supervision for nursing and health visiting. United Kingdom Central Council for Nursing, Midwifery and Health Visiting, London

Appendix: Supervisor self-assessment tool

Read the following statements and tick the box that you feel most accurately reflects the statement in relation to your own supervisory practice.

Questionnaire

Statement	Always	Sometimes	Never
1. I tend to suggest what is best for the supervisee before I know fully what is going on	❏	❏	❏
2. I start the session on time	❏	❏	❏
3. My feedback is based on observation of the supervisee in the session	❏	❏	❏
4. I avoid interactions that may cause conflict	❏	❏	❏
5. A supervisee has questioned my trust in a session before	❏	❏	❏
6. The supervisee evaluates how the session went	❏	❏	❏
7. The supervisee asks me to repeat questions I ask of them in a session	❏	❏	❏
8. I check on my supervisory performance with the supervisee during the session	❏	❏	❏
9. The clinical supervisor is in charge of the supervision session	❏	❏	❏
10. I try to understand how the supervisee feels before starting the session	❏	❏	❏
11. I accurately remember what has gone on during the session	❏	❏	❏
12. I frame what is going on for the supervisee using my own previous experiences	❏	❏	❏

Questionnaire (Cont.)

Statement	Always	Sometimes	Never
13. The supervisee does most of the talking in the supervision session	❏	❏	❏
14. The supervisee takes responsibility for recording what went on in supervision	❏	❏	❏
15. I actively try to use questions that will draw out the supervisee's clinical practice	❏	❏	❏
16. The session is ended on time	❏	❏	❏
17. I am able to apologise if necessary to the supervisee about my supervisory performance	❏	❏	❏
18. I find it difficult to concentrate on what the supervisee talks about in the session	❏	❏	❏
19. I give the supervisee a number of different options to consider about the situation they describe to me	❏	❏	❏
20. I ask questions in a way the supervisee can understand	❏	❏	❏
21. I ask the supervisee to summarise at the end what has gone on in the session	❏	❏	❏
22. I am clear about the purpose of clinical supervision	❏	❏	❏
23. The supervisee is relaxed during the session	❏	❏	❏
24. I am able to take on board constructive criticism by the supervisee on my performance as a clinical supervisor	❏	❏	❏
25. By listening to the supervisee's stories I can also learn about practice	❏	❏	❏
26. I find it straightforward enough to get the supervisee to talk at length about their practice	❏	❏	❏
27. I listen more than I talk in the session	❏	❏	❏
28. The supervisee helps me notice what is good about the supervision session	❏	❏	❏
29. I learn about aspects of myself as a supervisor during a session	❏	❏	❏
30. The supervision session can help me to reflect on my own practice	❏	❏	❏

Score each answer on the answer grid overleaf. Give yourself 3 marks for Always, 2 marks for Sometimes and 1 mark for Never. Total the scores for each baseline skill to work out your cumulative score. The maximum score for each of the six skills is 15, the minimum score is 5. Enter the total scores from each question into the table and see how you have done.

Answer grid

Baseline skills of the supervisor	Ability to open an emotional account with supervisee	Willingness to learn from supervision mutually with supervisee	Ability to be attentive to what is going on in the session	Ability to be use questions effectively to help supervisee notice 'self' in practice	Willingness to receive feedback from supervisee	Ability to summarise content of session
Question no. Your score	2	25	27	15	9	11
Question no. Your score	23	29	12	4	24	16
Question no. Your score	10	30	1	20	28	21
Question no. Your score	17	22	18	26	19	6
Question no. Your score	5	8	13	7	3	14
Maximum score	15	15	15	15	15	15
Your total score						
Minimum score	5	5	5	5	5	5

You have now formed your personal baseline from which to begin to think about gauging your performance as a clinical supervisor. On reflection, what sort of things have you learned and need to action in your clinical supervision?

You may wish to do this exercise again in 6 months' time to chart your progress as a clinical supervisor.

8 Supervisory approaches and styles

INTRODUCTION

Every clinical supervision relationship will bring together at least two different people. For clinical supervision to be effective, they will need to agree on what is going to happen in supervision sessions. There can be considerable conflict in a supervision situation where the supervisee and supervisor have not discussed beforehand how and in what way clinical supervision will be conducted. Supervisor and supervisee are both products of the organisational culture in which they work. This will also have a bearing on the approach to be adopted in their training packages, policies and protocols on clinical supervision.

In an ideal situation, the supervisee will have been able to choose the supervisor whom they consider will be most helpful to them. The element of choice is an important aspect in the continued development of clinical supervision. In reality, such a choice may be hard to come by until an adequate number of trained supervisors exist within an organisation. Clinical supervision has obvious financial as well as human resource implications for healthcare organisations investing heavily in an initiative that has yet to demonstrate its effectiveness in improving delivery of patient/client care.

This chapter will explore two mainstream approaches to clinical supervision and argue that, for most practitioners, reflection on practice is an approach that is becoming more familiar in everyday clinical practice. For more specialist practitioners, such as those in mental health, in learning disability or working closely with families, a more 'psychodynamic approach' may be more useful. Supervisory styles are also examined in relation to John Heron's (1989) Six Category Intervention Analysis, through which the reader can decide whether the process of supervision offered is more facilitative than authoritative.

TWO DIFFERENT APPROACHES TO CLINICAL SUPERVISION SESSIONS

Hawkins & Shohet (1994) offer two broad approaches to clinical supervision from the disciplines of counselling and psychotherapy, which have been widely publicised in the nursing literature (Faugier & Butterworth 1994, Farrington 1995, Hughes & Morcom 1996, Scanlon 1998). Good practice in supervision demands that both the supervisee and the supervisor are aware of the supervisory approaches to be used in the contractual phase, which may also include changing to a different approach at a later stage if both parties agree to this.

From the work of Hawkins & Shohet (1994), two broad approaches to supervision can be simplified as: Approach 1 – looking to the past to see the future, and Approach 2 – looking at the present to see the future (Box 8.1). In order for clinical supervision to be meaningful in nursing practice, both approaches are intended to offer ways of enhancing the individual supervisee's future clinical practice.

BOX 8.1	*Two approaches to supervision based on the intentions of the supervisor and supervisee*

Approach 1: Looking to the past to see the future – the supervisee's nursing practice is reported upon and reflected on in the supervision session

Possible foci of the supervision sessions:

- Reflection on the content of nursing practice in relation to the expressed needs of the patient/client, e.g. How well did the nurse get to know the patient/client?
- Exploration of the strategies and interventions used by the nurse to meet the patient/client needs, e.g. What choices were made by the nurse in clinical care and what were the consequences for the nurse and the patient/client?
- Exploration of the process or context of nursing in relation to where it was carried out, e.g. What were some of the challenges that the individual nurse had to face in delivering that nursing care?

Approach 2: Looking at the present to see the future – what goes on in the supervision session is reflected upon as an extension of what goes on in the supervisee's clinical practice

Possible foci of the supervision sessions:

- Finding out what baggage the supervisee carries about looking after a particular patient/client, e.g. exploring why the supervisee reacts to or feels in a particular way about a patient/client they are looking after (transference)?
- The here-and-now process of supervision as a mirror of what went on there and then in clinical practice, e.g. the relationship the supervisee has either consciously or unconsciously towards the supervisor parallels the hidden dynamics of the relationship between the nurses and the patient/client
- Sharing with the supervisee as the session unfolds what is going on or the images/feelings that are stirred up for the supervisor by the session (counter-transference). This forms the basis for learning opportunities for both parties in supervision, e.g. mutual sharing and exploration of supervision material

Approach 1 is similar to Schon's (1987) 'reflection on action' whereby the supervisee looks back with the clinical supervisor at significant events or practice stories that have happened in practice. The aim of this type of supervision is to learn by obtaining meaning from what happened and, with the help of the supervisor, to develop strategies for dealing with similar situations should they occur again. Much of this approach relies on the supervisee bringing in to the session practice events that have already happened. The content will usually be about:

- the supervisee in clinical practice
- the context of the supervisee's work
- the relationship between the supervisee and the patient/client(s).

Much of Approach 2 is similar to the interventions seen in a more formal counselling situation. It is a useful approach for nurses more used to working in a psychotherapeutic or analytical way, e.g. being non-judgemental and accepting of how the supervisee acts or 'reacts' in the session towards the supervisor. The emphasis is on trying to remain in touch with the present moment, sometimes referred to as the 'here and now', and help the supervisee interpret or acknowledge the significance of these events (Hughes & Morcom 1996, p. 48), rather than just reflecting on practice stories that happened some time ago.

Another important part of the 'here and now' process is the ability of the supervisor to recognise transference and countertransference occurring within supervision. A more detailed account of these can be found in O'Kelly (1998). Essentially, transference is an unconscious process by which the supervisee displaces feelings, thoughts and behaviours from a significant person in the past to a person in a current relationship, e.g. the clinical supervisor or a patient/client from clinical practice:

> **Supervisor:** 'I noticed that when you spoke about Chloe and her behaviour you became quite angry – is this how you feel about that behaviour of hers you were describing to me earlier?'
>
> **Supervisee:** 'I wasn't aware of being angry when I was talking about her ... what do you mean (raising voice)?'
>
> **Supervisor:** 'Are you aware that you are raising your voice with me now?'

Countertransference refers to any attitude and feeling that is experienced by a therapist towards the client in therapy that can hinder the therapeutic relationship. In supervision, countertransference can be a useful learning experience for the clinical supervisor if there is a mutual sharing or disclosure in supervision of what is being experienced in the 'here and now' experience of the clinical supervision session. Countertransference may occur in any supervisory relationship but may not be noticed unless the supervisor is purposely adopting this approach or at least is aware that such unconscious processes exist.

> **Supervisor:** 'I am becoming aware that I am getting distracted in the conversation we are having about Paul....'
>
> **Supervisee:** 'I'd noticed that as well – do you feel all right? Shall I open the window?'

Supervisor: 'To be honest, I think it's more to do with my annoyance that you do not seem to be noticing what is going on with Paul's situation ... perhaps it might be helpful if we explore this a bit more? I'm not intending to come across as uninterested, but I must admit I am starting to wander in our conversation ... what do you think?

The notion of the 'here and now' clinical supervision session as mirroring, or a parallel process to the supervisee's clinical practice (Dombeck & Brody 1995, Playle & Mullarkey 1998) can be particularly challenging for a supervisee who is not familiar with this approach and will require a high degree of support in the early stages as well as commitment to staying with this form of supervision. This approach does not rely solely on practice stories from the past. Instead the content will be about:

- the relationship between the supervisor and supervisee in the present
- actively noticing what aspects of the supervisory relationship mirror the supervisee's clinical practice.

Obviously this approach might seem 'different' or even not relevant to nurses working in a family planning clinic who attend for regular clinical supervision. Although it might be simply dismissed as 'analysis' that is more appropriate for mental health nursing, it is interesting to consider the possibilities for your own practice area. It might be interesting to discuss Box 8.2 as a staff group rather than just dismiss such an approach. Perhaps it may be an approach to adopt when you feel more confident in your own clinical supervision and wish to try this method out with a more specialist supervisor who has a background in mental health.

BOX 8.2	*An exercise exploring an alternative approach to clinical supervision for adult 'general' nurses*

- Can you think of a time when you really took an instant like, or dislike to somebody in clinical practice (e.g. a patient/client, student nurse, medical colleague or even your present clinical supervisor)?
- How likely is it that your reaction was due in part to that person reminding you of somebody significant to you in the past?
- What was it you liked or disliked?
- How did you behave towards that individual?
- What 'roadblocks' did you put in the way of effective communication between you and that person?
- What were the outcomes of your subsequent communication with that person?
- Might it have been different if this had been communicated to a clinical supervisor familiar with this type of supervisory technique?
- What might be the consequences of adult 'general' nurses adopting such an approach in their own clinical supervision practice?

IS CLINICAL SUPERVISION A THERAPY?

You might be forgiven for thinking that many of the approaches open to the supervisee and the supervisor in clinical supervision resemble some sort of personal therapy. However, the answer to the question 'Is clinical supervision a therapy?' has to be an emphatic 'No', although one must concede that looking at the skills used in disciplines such as counselling and psychotherapy can be another way of helping the supervisee to enhance their clinical performance.

Barker (1998, p. 67) in one of the most frequently referenced clinical supervision sources in nursing, makes the distinction between helpfulness and helping. He rightly suggests that nurses are portrayed traditionally as professionals who try to be helpful but invariably by intervening on behalf of the person in care. For example, nobody would argue about the helpful nature of the surgical nurse reassuring the anxious individual prior to elective surgery.

Helpfulness differs from helping, which is about that same surgical nurse arranging ways of promoting the growth and development of the same individual undergoing elective surgery. It is this aspect that is often missed in busy practice but forms the healing potential of the individual nurse, instead of just being a health 'caretaker' for the patient. Barker succinctly encapsulates the inherent dangers of a new clinical supervisor being helpful rather than *helping* in a supervision relationship, and this applies equally to all forms of relationship we have in clinical nursing practice: 'We should not lose sight of the fact that the more useful we are the more useless the person might become' (Barker 1998, p. 67).

Counselling or psychotherapy differs from clinical supervision in that it does not intentionally have as its prime focus the promotion of healing for the supervisee, although it must be acknowledged that some healing may take place (Deery & Corby 1996, p. 206). Dooher et al (1998, p. 36) distinguish between the expectations of a client in a therapy situation and those of the supervisee in clinical supervision. The former has therapeutic expectations of the counsellor while the latter requires guidance, support and the opportunity to reflect on their practice with another experienced professional.

Faugier (1998, p. 32), outlining the relationship component of her growth and support model of clinical supervision, leaves the reader in no doubt that clinical supervision is not therapy, but still recognises similarities in the supervisory relationship that contribute to the growth of the practitioner:

> The alliance between supervisor and supervisee is analogous to the therapeutic alliance defined as the bond of trust between nurse and patient which is necessary for the practice of high-quality nursing. By exploiting the emphasis on self-awareness issues in supervision, the supervisee may attempt to receive 'therapy' from the supervisor, thereby diverting the sessions into a situation where personal needs are the centre of attention. Similarly, supervisors may wish to demonstrate their own understanding of the human psyche and may be guilty of overanalysing the responses of the supervisee, which often leads to resentment and anger. All these relationship 'traps' do nothing to serve the real purpose of supervision, which is the promotion of learning about nursing, including some personal growth content.

Complete the diagram in Figure 8.1. Which statements do you feel apply to therapy, clinical supervision or both? Consider these in relation to your own expectations of clinical supervision as a supervisor or supervisee. This can be a useful exercise to bear in mind while clarifying in the first session what you expect clinical supervision to be, or not to be…. Is clinical supervision a therapy? That is the question!

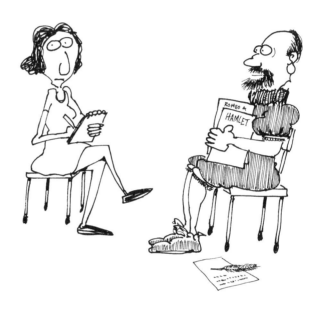

Accepting that clinical supervision is not a therapy but can be of a therapeutic nature for the supervisee, John Heron's Six Category Intervention Analysis (Heron 1989) is an example of how different counselling skills can be adapted by the clinical supervisor and how they can be a help as well as a hindrance in clinical supervision.

SIX WAYS A CLINICAL SUPERVISOR CAN HELP OR HINDER THE CLINICAL SUPERVISEE IN A SESSION

John Heron (1989) identified six verbal-counselling intervention(s) or styles, which can be used interchangeably and have an equal value, in that no one style is regarded as more important than the others. In clinical supervision training workshops, noticing how individuals interact helps supervisors recognise their favoured supervisory styles. The six categories of intervention are broadly grouped as either being of an authoritative or a facilitative nature (Box 8.3).

| Figure 8.1 | *Is clinical supervision a therapy?* |

	COUNSELLING	SUPERVISION	BOTH
Talking to a distressed person			
Assisting a person with a psychological disturbance			
Being interested in a person's personal development			
Giving information			
Creating a long term relationship			
Helping a person to reflect			
Giving feedback on performance			
Emphasising learning			
Helping a person express their feelings			
Being genuine with the person			
Clarifying what is happening for the other person			
Using a range of questions			
Work underpinned by humanistic theories about people			
Concerned with behaviours that may be of an unconscious origin			
Actively listening to what is being said			
Concern with the inner world of the person			
Being interested in what is being talked about			
Exploring solutions to 'problems'			
Being non-judgemental			

| BOX 8.3 | *Six possible interactions a clinical supervisor can have with the supervisee during a session* |

Authoritative interventions:

- Prescriptive: giving advice
- Informative: imparting information
- Confrontational: directly challenging

Facilitative interventions:

- Supportive: understanding and encouraging
- Cathartic: allowing the release of emotions
- Catalytic: encouraging deeper exploration

It is not difficult to see the potential differences between authoritative interventions or styles and facilitative interventions or styles, which are more suited to sustaining a successful supervisory relationship. The earlier discussion as to whether clinical supervision is a task or a process seems to fit the broad division in supervisor style. Clearly, the approach a supervisor is likely to use with the supervisee merits some discussion prior to clinical supervision. A relationship developing along the lines of the novice/expert model of supervised practice with more junior staff is less likely to be effective if both parties are already accountable for what they do in clinical practice.

The different styles of the supervisor can be seen more clearly using supervision examples to illustrate the different interventions.

Authoritative interventions

Prescriptive

Supervisee: 'I am at my wits end with that doctor: I've tried everything to make him see that the treatment cards need to be written up before the night staff come on duty.'

Supervisor: 'I think you should get the night staff to complain about him if you can't change the situation on days.'

Giving advice or recommending a course of action is something that tends to be popular in a busy ward situation. Often it is easier to tell a patient or a colleague what to do, but in supervision this type of intervention can give the impression that the supervisor knows best, even though clinical supervision is designed to be an 'enabling process'. Although there will be times when some form of direction is required, a supervisee can quickly learn that by asking the right questions they can get the supervisor to 'provide them with answers'. This can lead to the supervisee becoming dependent on the supervisor.

Informative

Supervisee: 'This is my first clinical supervision session....'

Supervisor: 'Well you will probably feel uncomfortable at first, most supervisees meeting their supervisor for the first time usually feel that way, but you'll get used to it.'

An informative style requires the supervisor to inform, or instruct the supervisee in some way. Many nurses will be familiar with 'teaching' things to students, patients or relatives. Again, overuse may lead to dependency and the supervisor 'overteaching' the supervisee by giving them information they could find out themselves. Clinical supervision is not 'I know all the answers because I am experienced' but a mutual sharing of expertise and experience. It can be useful to use in a concrete situation, however, e.g. 'Do you know Allan who works on the ward opposite? He's just taken up clinical supervision recently.'

Confrontational

Supervisor: 'I notice that when you talk about that patient you seem to raise your voice.'

Supervisee: 'Oh ... er ... do I? ... Well, it's a bit noisy outside this room!'

Supervisor: 'I've closed the window ... but I'd still like you to think about why, with that particular patient?'

This intervention challenges the supervisee to look at some action or behaviour noted by the supervisor. The supervisee can often be taken aback not only by what has been said, but also how it has been said. Often, the supervisor has brought the issue into the supervisee's conscious awareness for the first time and they need time to consider their response. Unless handled with care, far from being illuminating and raising awareness, it can also be perceived as the supervisor being too 'aggressive' by pushing the supervisee too quickly. This can have the effect of making the supervisee more defensive about what they do or say and less open in communicating with the supervisor in the future.

Facilitative interventions

Supportive

Supervisee: 'I must be honest, I was unsure of what the medication was for – I had never heard of it before.... The rest of the patients were a bit uptight with me for making them wait, but I needed to read up a bit before I gave it.'

Supervisor: 'I can understand your concerns and why you acted like that ... you must have felt awkward about the patients getting so impatient with you, but it appears to me that you acted in a safe and professional manner as regards the medication.'

This intervention requires the skills of active listening by the supervisor in order to comment on what has been said and encourage the supervisee in some way. This might be to support an action taken by them. Although being supportive may seem obvious, it is important for the supervisor to listen in order to understand what is going on for the supervisee so that they can decide whether a supportive intervention is appropriate. Badly used, such an intervention can be perceived by the supervisee as patronising rather than supportive. As nurses, we are often accused of reassuring or lessening the anxiety of someone without fully knowing what it is we are reassuring – because we were 'too busy' to find out.

Cathartic

Supervisee: 'It was absolutely dreadful – it had been a nightmare of a shift with three admissions that evening ... when I finally managed to go back to check on Mr Brock I found that he had slipped away.... I'm sorry.' (apologising to the supervisor)

Supervisor: 'It's OK to feel the way you do, Teresa, take your time.' (short pause)

Supervisee: '"It's OK" – what do you mean, "It's OK?" Because of me he died alone! I would hate that to happen to me ... that's what I'm there for, isn't it?... but I was so bloody busy with other things ... that ... that I forgot him!' (supervisee begins to cry)

These interventions allow the supervisee to release emotions associated with the situation that is being discussed. In many cases it may need 'permission' for this release of emotion (catharsis) to occur. Crying and being angry in a session are two examples of cathartic activities that can be facilitated by giving space, as in silence, or verbally giving permission for the supervisee to become emotional. A moral dimension enters the relationship if the supervisor intentionally 'pushes' the supervisee into releasing feelings when they are not ready or are unwilling to do so. The supervisee should decide, not the supervisor, if and when such emotional release should occur. Inexperienced supervisors may also feel inadequate because they do not know what to do in such situations. A way to deal with such uncertainty can be to try to reduce your own anxiety by reducing the supervisee's feelings, e.g. 'Oh, don't be so silly, it wasn't your fault – you said you'd had a nightmare shift!'

Catalytic

> **Supervisee:** 'I couldn't believe it – only last week I felt that I wanted to leave, especially after the row I had with the charge nurse when he cancelled the staff meeting about the poor evaluations we received from the last batch of students, and since that point I don't seem to have put a foot wrong with him ... he has been really good to me and let me have a couple of hours in his office to rethink the student induction programme.'

> **Supervisor:** 'I think that's a really useful thing to look at today – in what ways do you think the conflict with the charge nurse contributed to what has happened this week? Is it you or the charge nurse who has changed?... What is so different for you?'

Interventions such as these encourage the supervisee to draw out and explore issues at a deeper level than just superficially describing what went on. Part of being reflective is the ability to allow the supervisee to describe the situation in their own words before attempting to find out why or how. Such interventions require a particular type of explorative questioning that might be seen as inquisitorial or prying. It can be useful to keep to more open questions, or questions that the supervisor starts and allows the supervisee to complete, e.g. 'Am I right in thinking that the conflict seems to have altered your practice?' In the case above, too many catalytic or open questions can cause confusion for the supervisee and make them lose track of how they were feeling before.

You may wish to observe interactions in clinical practice and notice not just the intervention(s) used in a conversation, but the outcome for the overall conversation, whether in the coffee room or during a ward round involving patients/clients and staff.

In what way do you think having an understanding of the six categories of intervention might help you in clinical supervision? Compare your own ideas to Box 8.4.

BOX 8.4	*Ways in which Six Category Intervention Analysis might be helpful in clinical supervision*

Six Category Intervention Analysis can:

- help you to appreciate the wide range of possible interventions in supervision
- heighten your awareness of the type of interventions you tend to use most
- challenge you to consider more facilitative approaches in supervision
- encourage consideration of how different types of question elicit particular responses
- allow you to intentionally use different types of communication in the one-to-one situation
- make you aware of alternatives to your normal responses in practice.

This chapter has presented a number of different approaches that are already used in health related disciplines other than nursing – counselling, psychotherapy, midwifery and social work. It is important to note that no one approach is right or wrong for a discipline as diverse as nursing. Much of the clamour by practitioners in clinical supervision workshops is asking 'How should we go about it?', as if there might be some magical right way for everyone.

In some respects, there are similarities between such a question and the supervisee asking, or relying on the clinical supervisor to indicate, how supervision is done. The uncertainty for the new supervisee (or the inexperienced supervisor) about to how to 'do' supervision can be viewed as developmental. The supervisee quickly learns that the supervisor is not a 'personal adviser', and then begins to explore ways to make supervision most effective for them and for their practice, and, more importantly, to contribute to their patients' and clients' wellbeing.

In my view it would be very wrong at such an early stage in the development of clinical supervision in nursing to dismiss any particular approach in favour of another. It is very possible to negotiate supervision in such a way that it allows a change to a different approach at a later time.

The answer to the mystery lies in disseminating what supervisees and supervisors consider to be good supervision. In other words, the truth is probably already out there, but we must in the first instance be guided by other disciplines more experienced in supervision and then adapt their approaches to our own practice situations. In this way, clinical supervision, far from being imposed, will emerge from within nursing.

Clinical supervision is a complex delivery service that involves a willingness to change the culture of nursing's 'work' environment into a more supportive learning environment. This means that finding regular space, e.g. every month, at what Sams (1996) calls the reflective oasis of clinical supervision, is just as important as doing the work. Learning in clinical supervision is also about taking a few risks in order to become more creative in how we approach nursing work. The diversity of different approaches can only help in accommodating the needs of those engaged in supervision, as well as offering alternative ways of seeing clinical practice with the intention of enhancing the care delivered.

On reflection ... chapter summary

What are the key elements of this chapter?

- Clinical supervision approaches should be agreed beforehand

- The organisational culture will have a bearing on the supervisory approach adopted in clinical practice

- Clinical supervision approaches can involve looking back on practice or staying with the present to influence future practice

- Although clinical supervision is not a therapy it can have a therapeutic effect on supervisees

- The ways in which we communicate in clinical supervision will have a direct effect on the outcome of clinical supervision in practice

So what difference does this make to the way I am operating my clinical/ supervisory practice?

Now what actions will need to be taken as a result of my reflections?

REFERENCES

Barker P 1998 Psychiatric nursing. In: Butterworth T, Faugier J, Burnard P (eds) Clinical supervision and mentorship in nursing, 2nd edn. Stanley Thornes, Cheltenham, UK, ch 5, p 66–80

Deery R, Corby D 1996 A case for clinical supervision in midwifery. In: Kirkham M (ed) Supervision of midwives. Books for Midwives Press, Hale, ch 14

Dombeck MT, Brody SL 1995 Clinical supervision: a three way mirror. Archives of Psychiatric Nursing 9(1): 3–10

Dooher J, Fowler J, Phillips A, North R, Wells A 1998 Demystifying clinical supervision. In: Fowler J (ed) The handbook of clinical supervision – your questions answered. Quay Books, Salisbury, ch 1, p 1–46

Farrington A 1995 Models of clinical supervision. British Journal of Nursing 4(15): 876–878

Faugier J 1998 The supervisory relationship. In: Butterworth T, Faugier J, Burnard P (eds) Clinical supervision and mentorship in nursing, 2nd edn. Stanley Thornes, Cheltenham, ch 2, p 19–36

Faugier J, Butterworth T 1994 Clinical supervision: a position paper (given at the first Department of Health Conference on Clinical Supervision in Birmingham). School of Nursing Studies, University of Manchester, Manchester, p. 1–60

Hawkins P, Shohet R 1994 Supervision in the helping professions. Open University Press, Milton Keynes

Heron J 1989 The facilitators handbook. Kogan Page, London

Hughes R, Morcom C 1996 Clinical supervision – distance learning package. Warrington Community Health Care (NHS) Trust, Warrington

O'Kelly G 1998 Countertransference in the nurse–patient relationship: a review of the literature. Journal of Advanced Nursing 28(2): 391–397

Playle JF, Mullarkey K 1998 Parallel process in clinical supervision: enhancing learning and providing support. Nurse Education Today (18): 558–566

Sams DA 1996 Clinical supervision: an oasis for practice. British Journal of Community Health Nursing 1(2): 88–91

Scanlon C 1998 Towards effective training of
clinical supervisors. In: Bishop V (ed)
Clinical supervision in practice: some
questions, answers and guidelines.

Macmillan/Nursing Times Research
Publications, London, ch 7, p 143–162
Schon D 1987 The reflective practitioner.
Avebury Publishing, Aldershot

3 THE CHALLENGE OF CLINICAL SUPERVISION

The purpose of Part 3 is to:

- assist the reader to become more self-regulating about what goes on during the clinical supervision sessions and more aware of how difficulties can arise and, more importantly, how they can be avoided

- foster an enquiring approach towards not only how effective clinical supervision can enhance the individual practitioner and the organisation, but also the ways in which clients and patients benefit from nurses being collectively engaging in clinical supervision

- offer some practical guidance as to how clinical supervision can be started and sustained in busy clinical practice

- openly invite practitioners already engaging in clinical supervision, in whatever practice environment, to discover ways and means of helping others by disseminating some of their own successes and difficulties in getting clinical supervision off the ground.

Barriers to effective communication in clinical supervision

INTRODUCTION

Much of the literature on clinical supervision to date has attempted to clarify what clinical supervision in nursing is and how it can become a reality. Debate also centres on the potential value of clinical supervision for individual practitioners, their patients and clients, and the organisation within which they work.

In contrast, books on clinical supervision by other health-related disciplines in which it has been a feature for some years (e.g. social work, counselling, psychotherapy and mental health nursing) reflect ways in which the supervision encounter can be a difficult and challenging journey for the supervisor as well as the supervisee.

What is communicated 'over the clinical supervision coffee table' between supervisor and supervisee can be quite different from what is really going on beneath it! Ineffective communication can be employed by either the supervisor or supervisee and become a source of dissatisfaction and conflict, ultimately leading to avoidance.

The development of effective communication strategies between supervisors and supervisees is a key aspect of training workshops in clinical supervision. By adapting aspects of transactional analysis theory, this chapter intends to help the clinical supervisor and supervisee to become more aware of the different psychological processes that can go on in the clinical supervision relationship. In doing so, it will also help the clinical supervisor formulate some useful agenda items for their own supervision, as well as offer insight to both, on how to maximise the use of 'talking time' in clinical practice.

WHO'S IN CHARGE WHEN YOU COMMUNICATE WITH OTHERS?

Bailey & Baillie (1996) suggest that effective communication and the development of interpersonal relationships are essential features in the development of skilled and competent nursing practitioners. The same is also true for a successful clinical supervision partnership. They cite Eric Berne's theory (Berne 1968) of personality and systematic psychotherapy, commonly referred to as transactional analysis, as a useful tool for illustrating common communication behaviours that can be observed in clinical practice. It is important to be clear that, in the context of clinical supervision, transactional analysis is simply a tool for exploring the different patterns of communication that can arise in the supervisory encounter. Each of the patterns outlined also occurs in everyday communication and should not be viewed as simply right or wrong, or good or bad. Although clinical supervision is not psychotherapy for nurses, transactional analysis offers an alternative way of viewing how we communicate with each other.

Read the History Box involving Eilish the senior staff nurse.
   Now consider the five different responses to what has happened.
   Which of the five responses might you have used to Raj, if it had been you in a similar situation?
   Are there any responses that Eilish or Raj use that you would say are:
a) definitely you in practice; b) definitely not you in practice?

History Box   The ward clerk has noticed that the consultant surgeon and her entourage have just arrived to do the ward round on the unit opposite. She informs Eilish, the senior staff nurse, who suddenly remembers that Mr Jones's wound drain should have been removed the day before. Eilish asks Raj, the student nurse, to wheel Mr Jones into the treatment room while she prepares the trolley. A few minutes later, Raj backs into the treatment room with Mr Jones, crashing into Eilish's prepared dressing trolley and sending the contents over the floor and bed.

Response 1

Eilish: 'Oh you stupid idiot, Raj! How many times have I told you to look where you're going? Just wait until the consultant sees what you've done!'

Raj: 'Oh, I'm sorry, Eilish (wishing the ground would swallow him up and thinking of his placement report next week) – why does this always happen to me?'

Response 2

Eilish: 'Oh! ... are you OK, you two?... No bones broken, are there?'

Raj: 'No, I don't think so, but I gave my elbow a bit of a knock, though.'

Response 3

Eilish: 'Just forget the mess, Raj, the consultant will be here in a minute.... Can you lay up a fresh trolley for drain removal so I can keep these gloves on? We can both clear up the room after the drain has come out.'

Raj: 'I saw Samantha laying up a trolley – I'll borrow her one and be back in a jiffy.... Sorry about that, Mr Jones, you should see me at the end of a night shift!'

Response 4

Eilish: 'Oh, now look what you've done!' (bursting into tears and throwing the gloves across at Raj)

Raj: (ducking the thrown gloves and stooping down on to his hands and knees) 'I really didn't mean it – I'll clear the mess up for you!'

Response 5

Eilish: (feeling a bit panicky) 'Quick, get some more equipment from the storeroom, Raj, so we can get this done before the consultant gets here – go the long way round to avoid meeting her.'

Raj: 'OK – I'll hurry up and get the others to keep an eye out for us!'

Berne (1968, p. 23) suggested that when we communicate to others we can act, feel and think in any one of three ways or ego states. Stewart & Joines (1987, p. 21), in a very readable text on transactional analysis (TA), subdivide the three ego states into five different communication patterns (Figure 9.1).

| **Figure 9.1** | *Five different communication patterns or ego states* |

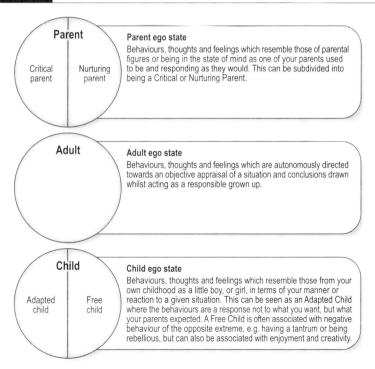

Parent
Critical parent | Nurturing parent

Parent ego state
Behaviours, thoughts and feelings which resemble those of parental figures or being in the state of mind as one of your parents used to be and responding as they would. This can be subdivided into being a Critical or Nurturing Parent.

Adult

Adult ego state
Behaviours, thoughts and feelings which are autonomously directed towards an objective appraisal of a situation and conclusions drawn whilst acting as a responsible grown up.

Child
Adapted child | Free child

Child ego state
Behaviours, thoughts and feelings which resemble those from your own childhood as a little boy, or girl, in terms of your manner or reaction to a given situation. This can be seen as an Adapted Child where the behaviours are a response not to what you want, but what your parents expected. A Free Child is often associated with negative behaviour of the opposite extreme, e.g. having a tantrum or being rebellious, but can also be associated with enjoyment and creativity.

While these examples are an oversimplification of modern TA, they do offer some clues to ways in which grown-up people can communicate with each other based on the recognition of ego states. When TA is used as a psychotherapy, each of the five elements is said to be an aspect of a person's personality.

Effective communication in clinical supervision requires both parties in the relationship to regularly consider this question, in order to ensure that what is happening over the clinical supervision coffee table accurately reflects what is going on beneath it.

The use of TA in clinical supervision is to analyse not personalities, but different communication behaviours involving the supervisor and supervisee. In training workshops or events, it can be insightful to analyse the communication behaviours of the supervisee or supervisor in relation to the Parent–Adult–Child framework that TA adopts.

It is useful to note that Parent and Child behaviours, feelings and thoughts emerge from *your* distant past: in Child they are a replay of *your own* child-hood responses, in Parent they are a copy of *your* parents' own responses to you. It is only when in Adult that you can respond to situations in the present time, using all *your* known resources as a grown-up. It is this final state, being a grown-up and responding in an Adult ego state, that becomes the bedrock of a successful clinical supervision relationship.

Some of the more observable communication patterns using TA are summarised in Box 9.1, but you can probably think of many more to include.

BOX 9.1	*Some observable communication patterns using transactional analysis*

Parent	
Critical Parent	**Nurturing Parent**
Behaviours	*Behaviours*
Criticises	Protects
Commands	Comforts
Dictates	Helps
Attitude	*Attitude*
Judgemental	Understanding
Moralistic	Caring
Authoritarian	Giving
Smothering	
Words often used	*Words often used*
Must, always, ought, right, wrong, don't	Well done, good, love, help, leave it to me
Voice	*Voice*
Critical	Loving
Condescending	Comforting
Sarcastic	Helpful
Firm	Sweet
Domineering	Passive

| BOX 9.1 Cont. | *Some observable communication patterns using transactional analysis* |

Adult

Behaviours: Enquires, Analyses, Tests out reasons, Gives and receives information, Remains in the present

Attitude: Interested, Observant, Rational, Evaluates

Words often used: How, What, Why, Likely, Consider

Voice: Calm, Clear, Questioning, Precise, Monotone

Child

Adapted Child	Free Child
Behaviours	*Behaviours*
Reacts	Feels
Submits	Expresses
Accepts	
Rebels	
Attitude	*Attitude*
Compliant	Curious
Ashamed	Fun-loving
Apologetic	Changeable
Demanding	Self-centred
Well mannered	
Words often used	*Words often used*
Can't	Now
Try	Want
Sorry	Fun
Thank you	Joke
Voice	*Voice*
Whingeing	Free
Defiant	Loud
Placating	Energetic
Moaning	Happy
Demanding	

Take another look at some of the observable communication patterns in Box 9.1. Are there particular ego states, Parent, Adult or Child, that you tend to use more in clinical practice with, for instance:

■ the ward clerk?
■ your line manager?
■ the general practitioner/consultant?
■ the student nurse?

How much of your communication behaviour with others in clinical practice takes place in an Adult ego state?

Is it possible that you could change the way you communicate with these people – if so, how: what would need to happen?

Stewart & Joines (1987, p. 19) summarise the Parent–Adult–Child model of transactional analysis in the following way: 'When I am in Adult I will often be thinking. In Child I will often be into feelings. And when I am in Parent, I will often be making value judgements.'

Many of the definitions of clinical supervision seen in earlier chapters suggest engaging in a process that takes place within the confines of the relationship, or interactions between the clinical supervisor and supervisee. Kadushin (1992, p. 240), in an authoritative text on social work supervision, unintentionally evokes transactional analysis as a way of viewing how the clinical supervision relationship can also become a barrier to effectively communicating with each other.

'The supervisory relationship is an intense, intimate, personalised situation that has considerable emotional charge.... The supervisor–supervisee relationship evokes the parent–child relationship and, as such, may reactivate anxiety associated with this earlier relationship. If the supervisor is a potential parent surrogate, fellow supervisees are potential siblings competing for the affectionate responses of the parent.'

Obviously, the intention while in clinical supervision is to remain an Adult in the present, using what resources one has as a grown-up, rather than communicating in a Child or Parent ego state. This is more difficult to achieve than might perhaps be thought, as all psychologically healthy individuals switch between all the ego states in normal communication with others. Much depends on the context of the communication.

In reality, all of us can change between them all during a conversation. What is important to note is that, although we may have favoured ways of communicating with certain people, we all have a choice to stay as we are or change our communication transactions.

THE USE OF TRANSACTIONS IN THE CLINICAL SUPERVISION ENCOUNTER

Berne (1968, p. 28) describes a unit of social intercourse or communication as a transaction. In a single unit of communication, one person will stimulate a communication with another person, e.g. acknowledging them with 'Hello'. In turn, the second person will respond to the communication stimulus offered, by saying 'Hello' back, or choose not to. There are three different types of transaction that can all elicit different responses:

- Complementary transactions
- Crossed transactions
- Hidden transactions.

Complementary transactions

When transactions are complementary, communication will continue indefinitely providing that there are no surprises in the responses and that they are appropriate to what is being asked. Complementary transactions often occur when both participants adopt the same ego state, as outlined in Box 9.1, e.g. Parent–Parent, Child–Child or Adult–Adult. Consider the following transactions in a clinical supervision encounter.

Parent–Parent

Supervisor: 'Did those new doctors prevent you from getting away from the unit again?'

Supervisee: 'Yes, they're an awful bunch we've got this time, aren't they?'

The understanding Parent criticises the doctors on the ward for the supervisee's lateness, the response could equally be that of a sarcastic Parent.

Adult–Adult

Supervisor: 'Thank you for being on time today – we're a bit busy on the unit.'

Supervisee: 'That's OK, we had agreed this time the last time we met.'

Both have exchanged 'here and now' information using Adult words to each other. A third party could have also observed appropriate voices and gestures to each other in an Adult manner.

Child–Child

Supervisor: 'Come and sit down and let's have a cigarette together.'

Supervisee: 'We really shouldn't, in here, but no one will know.'

Both exchanges could be viewed as naughty children taking advantage of a supervision situation to escape from clinical practice and engage in deviant behaviour.

All the above exchanges could continue indefinitely. Each part of the transaction is met with the expected type of response, which keeps the communication flowing. Communication does not always require both parties to be in the same ego state for it to continue to be complementary and keep moving. Consider the following Parent–Child and Child–Parent transactions:

Critical Parent–Adapted Child

Supervisor: 'You're ten minutes late for supervision again ... do you think I have nothing else to do?'

Supervisee: (cowering and blushing) 'Sorry! I promise not to be late again – can we still spend the time together?'

Adapted Child–Nurturing Parent

Supervisor: (arriving 10 minutes late hot and flustered) 'I'm sorry to keep you waiting – I couldn't park!'

Supervisee: 'Don't worry, I often find parking a problem.... I've made some coffee for you.'

Crossed transactions

The previous type of communication illustrated how, when transactions are complementary, conversations will continue. But how many times have you in conversation heard or used the expressions 'I think we are talking at cross purposes' or 'I think our lines are crossed'? Crossed transactions occur as a result of not getting the expected response from the ego state we were trying to communicate with. The only way to continue with the conversation is for one or both individuals to shift ego states. Let us turn the previous example of a complementary transaction between the supervisor and supervisee into a crossed one.

Adult–Critical Parent (unexpected response)

Supervisor: 'Thank you for being on time today – we're a bit busy on the unit.'

Supervisee: (angry) 'You're a fine one to preach about being on time – it's you that's normally late!'

A crossed transaction has obviously occurred between the supervisor and supervisee. The response is not complementary and is not expected by the supervisor initiating the transaction.

What might be your next response as a clinical supervisor – Parent, Adult or Child?

How likely is it that your response to the supervisee will continue or end the conversation?

It is quite likely that you chose to adopt a more defensive Child mode to rescue the situation and complement the Critical Parent response of the supervisee, e.g. by apologising for your previous lateness. It is also possible that you view your main source of defence as verbally attacking the supervisee for their outburst to regain some control of the situation.

Crossed transactions need not always be a negative aspect of communication. A clinical supervisor can purposely use crossed transactions to reduce superficial and unproductive supervisory conversations with the supervisee. Crossed transactions can also be used to challenge aspects of the supervisee's clinical practice.

While retreating to a Child or Parent ego state might rescue the situation for you as a supervisor and return to more complementary transactions with the supervisee, in the above scenario it is unlikely to be productive. The supervisor can therefore elect to remain in a crossed Adult ego state and aim to bring a complementary transaction by appealing to the Adult in the supervisee.

Adult–Critical Parent (unexpected response)

Supervisor: (entering hurriedly 5 minutes late) 'Thank you for being on time today – we're a bit busy on the unit.'

Supervisee: (angry) 'You're a fine one to preach about being on time – it's you that's normally late!'

Adult–Adapted child (altered response)

Supervisor: (allowing some silence so that the supervisee can calm down) Thank you for bringing up my previous lateness intruding into what amounts to your time also – I understand why you're angry with me.'

Supervisee: (some initial embarrassment and unable to look the supervisor in the eye) 'I've had a hellish shift and I wanted to take some time owing today instead of coming to supervision … (begins to cry) … and then you weren't here….'

Adult–Adult (expected response)

Supervisor: 'Would you prefer to cancel the session, as you now have the opportunity to take your time back?'

Supervisee: 'No, let's continue with the session – I'd like to talk about what went on today.'

Adult–Adult (more productive conversation)

Supervisor: 'Just before we get into that, I'm concerned, as you are, with my lateness – is it possible we could renegotiate the times we meet?'

Supervisee: 'OK … I'm sorry I let fly at you. Perhaps my bad shift has had a positive effect!'

Adult–Adult

Supervisor: 'Yes, it's highlighted for me to do something about my lateness and perhaps, for you, how factors outside supervision can contribute to what goes on within it.'

Supervisee: 'That's supervision … we can both learn from one another.'

Hidden transactions

Hidden transactions are the double messages that may be contained in the communication one is having with another person. In other words, what is being communicated over the supervision coffee table can be quite different from what is going on beneath the supervision coffee table between the supervisee and supervisor!

Clues to hidden transactions can often be observed not just by listening to what is being said but by noting how the message is conveyed to you non-verbally. To communicate effectively with each other, we have to learn to distinguish between what is being communicated and how it is being said.

Box 9.2 contains a list of observable behaviours based on Ewles & Simnett's (1996, p. 150) categories of non-verbal communication.

You may wish to consider how these normal non-verbal behaviours could present as double messages or hidden transactions in your clinical practice. Are you aware of using hidden transactions yourself, or when someone is using them with you? In clinical supervision they can often be a sign that the relationship is undergoing some difficulties, or a marker of the stage the relationship is really at.

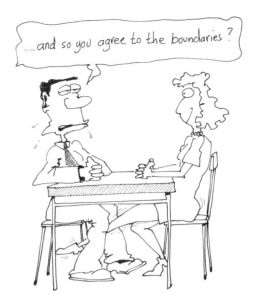

BOX 9.2	*Some categories of non-verbal communication*

- **Bodily contact** – shaking hands, putting an arm around a person's shoulder
- **Proximity** – the amount of space between the two people
- **Orientation** – the layout of the supervision venue
- **Level** – the difference in height level between the two people
- **Posture** – the position each person takes up with respect to the other
- **Physical appearance** – how the two people appear to one another
- **Facial expression** – indicating happiness, sadness, level of interest
- **Hand and head movements** – fidgeting, stress, relaxed
- **Direction of gaze and eye contact** – demonstrating interest or lack of interest, particularly when associated with listening
- **Tone and timing of speech** – a raised or quiet voice, persistent interrupting
- **Listening** – accurately recalling aspects of what is being said

How hidden transactions can relate to different stages of the clinical supervision relationship

Of the three transactions described, hidden transactions are potentially the most damaging way of communicating in clinical supervision. Kadushin (1992, p. 280) refers to such hidden transactions as 'defensive adjustments to the threats and anxieties that the supervisory situation poses for both supervisees and supervisors'. This is also suggestive that both parties, not just the supervisee, can indulge in such defensive strategies limiting effective communication.

Dolley et al (1998, p. 120) make a useful contribution to clinical supervision by suggesting that the clinical supervision relationship can pass through five developmental stages (Figure 9.2).

| Figure 9.2 | *Five stages of the clinical supervision relationship* (Dolley et al 1998) |

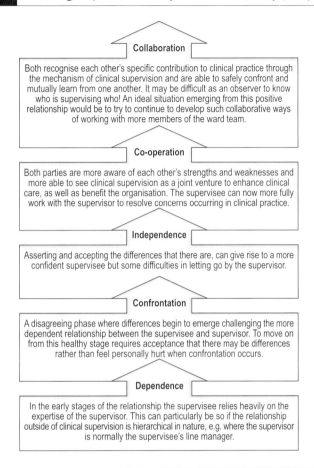

Collaboration

Both recognise each other's specific contribution to clinical practice through the mechanism of clinical supervision and are able to safely confront and mutually learn from one another. It may be difficult as an observer to know who is supervising who! An ideal situation emerging from this positive relationship would be to try to continue to develop such collaborative ways of working with more members of the ward team.

Co-operation

Both parties are more aware of each other's strengths and weaknesses and more able to see clinical supervision as a joint venture to enhance clinical care, as well as benefit the organisation. The supervisee can now more fully work with the supervisor to resolve concerns occurring in clinical practice.

Independence

Asserting and accepting the differences that there are, can give rise to a more confident supervisee but some difficulties in letting go by the supervisor.

Confrontation

A disagreeing phase where differences begin to emerge challenging the more dependent relationship between the supervisee and supervisor. To move on from this healthy stage requires acceptance that there may be differences rather than feel personally hurt when confrontation occurs.

Dependence

In the early stages of the relationship the supervisee relies heavily on the expertise of the supervisor. This can particularly be so if the relationship outside of clinical supervision is hierarchical in nature, e.g. where the supervisor is normally the supervisee's line manager.

Looking more critically at the five stages of the clinical supervision relationship can help to understand some of the reasons why both supervisor or supervisee may engage in hidden transactions with one another. Noticing them and challenging their use can transform the clinical supervision relationship, providing both parties are willing to openly communicate with each other in Adult ego states after they are discovered!

Using the descriptions of the stages of the clinical supervision relationship given in Figure 9.2, at what developmental stage do you consider your own clinical supervision to be, as either a clinical supervisor or a supervisee?

Write short notes on the following, as an aide-memoire for your next supervision session:

- Two **hidden** transactions (only you are aware of them) that you employed as a supervisee with your supervisor or, alternatively, as a supervisor with your supervisee
- What were your reasons for doing so?
- Was the outcome you hoped for in using the hidden transaction achieved?

Compare your responses to the same exercise carried out independently by Jocelyn, a clinical supervisor (Figure 9.3), and her supervisee Kim (Figure 9.4). This became the focus for a clinical supervision session aimed at identifying what stage their clinical supervision relationship was and how they could both get more from their time spent together.

Figure 9.3	*Hidden transactions occurring between Jocelyn, a clinical supervisor, and Kim, her supervisee*

Using the descriptions of the stages of the clinical supervision relationship given in Figure 9.2, what developmental stage do you consider your own clinical supervision to be, as a clinical supervisor?

Independence – I encourage Kim to be assertive about the way practice should be.

Write short notes on the following, as an aide-memoire for your next supervision session:

- Two **hidden** transactions (only you are aware of them) that you employed as a supervisor with your supervisee

1. *I summed the session up a few minutes earlier than usual because I needed to be at a meeting and Kim seemed to be rambling on a bit and not listening to what I was saying.*

2. *I like Kim a lot, and on a couple of occasions have gone along with what she has been saying although I haven't in fact agreed with her.*

- What were your reasons for doing so?

1. *I didn't want to let Kim know I wanted to leave early because I knew she had had to make an effort to be there and didn't want to disappoint her.*

2. *I find it difficult being assertive with Kim because we are friends and I don't want to hurt her feelings – after all, she's accountable for her own practice.*

- Was the outcome you hoped for in using the hidden transaction achieved?

Yes and no – although I succeeded in what I intended, I wish I could be more frank with her, but am not sure how to be.

Figure 9.4	*Hidden transactions occurring between Kim, a supervisee, and Jocelyn, her clinical supervisor*

Using the descriptions of the stages of the clinical supervision relationship given in Figure 9.2, what developmental stage do you consider your own clinical supervision to be, as a supervisee?

Dependence – I try to wind Jocelyn up for her to challenge what I do, but in some ways she's a bit too soft.

Write short notes on the following, as an aide-memoire for your next supervision session:

■ Two **hidden** transactions (only you are aware of them) that you employed as a supervisee with your supervisor

1. *I sometimes purposely have used our friendship to avoid exploring why I did something a particular way. I can usually get round this by buttering her up a bit.*

2. *I've found that, if I keep the discussion going about something Jocelyn doesn't know too much about, like pain management, I can avoid talking about the real issues.*

■ What were your reasons for doing so?

1. *I find clinical supervision difficult when I have to explain why, at times, I have been so stupid in practice, so it's better not to go down too deep into it.*

2. *I find it easier to have a conversation in general terms about what's going on in practice – I suppose I'm a bit afraid that I might not like what I hear Jocelyn saying about my practice.*

■ Was the outcome you hoped for in using the hidden transaction achieved?

Yes and no – although I can usually get around Jocelyn not to disclose too much about myself I'm beginning to wonder what the point of clinical supervision is and what Jocelyn is trying to do as a clinical supervisor. If it carries on like this for much longer I'll seriously have to question why we are both wasting practice time.

Commentary   Clearly there is a mutual respect for each other in clinical supervision, but to the point of collusion. From the hidden transactions between Jocelyn and Kim a pattern of clinical supervision emerges. They both find it difficult. Kim finds it difficult to disclose aspects of clinical practice, instead preferring to talk in general and superficial terms with Jocelyn. Jocelyn is unable to assert herself with Kim, her supervisee and friend, preferring to believe that Kim is accountable for clinical practice (which she is), and avoids any communication that might cause conflict or damage the friendship. *(continued over)*

> They differ as to what stage they believe the supervisory relationship between them is at. It is likely that they are both dependent on one another. In some respects, the hidden transactions undertaken by Kim serve both in the relationship. Kim avoids having to disclose too much by flattery and some emotional blackmail and, by not challenging this, Jocelyn avoids having to be assertive and cause any conflict between them. A point of note is that both are unhappy with the clinical supervision relationship but are not open and honest enough with each other to say so. Worse still, Kim is beginning to find that she is not getting much out of clinical supervision and is perhaps considering ways of avoiding it.

Clearly, hidden transactions between the supervisee and supervisor are an ineffective form of communication. They are a maladaptive response to actual or potential stresses associated with the new roles being adopted in clinical supervision, often as a result of inexperience (Box 9.3).

One of the consequences of ineffective communication in clinical supervision is that, rather than enhancing clinical practice, sessions become unpredictable and cause anxiety to both participants. This can further lead to a belief that clinical supervision is not as important as doing the work and to employing avoidance tactics so as not to have to attend. This can be particularly demoralising for staff who have spent time, money and effort in getting the system off the ground, along with all the other expectations of clinical supervision in practice.

TOWARDS MORE EFFECTIVE COMMUNICATION IN CLINICAL SUPERVISION – BEING ADULTS AS GROWN-UPS?

Becoming aware of hidden transactions can be a useful learning experience for the supervisee and supervisor. Once hidden transactions become evident and can be tackled in a more open way, the clinical supervision relationship can be transformed into what it should really be – a means of supporting and developing the practitioner to deliver quality care through critical reflection on practice. Sometimes one has to accept that there is an obvious mismatch – at one extreme the relationship may be devoid of trust or at the other it may be so collusive that nothing is being achieved. Both, Inskipp & Proctor (1995) rightly suggest, are clear indicators for changing supervisor.

In some circumstances, where there is very little choice of supervisor (or supervisee), the process may benefit from having a third party to give some feedback on what is going on in clinical supervision sessions. Sometimes just talking to other supervisors or supervisees may also be useful. Ideally, any policy or protocol for clinical supervision should include a mechanism whereby supervisors can discuss their supervisory practice in an informal or formal setting with other supervisors.

This chapter has focused on some of the communication difficulties that can be experienced in clinical supervision. Many of these can be reduced by the participants being open enough to air their concerns within the session. Sometimes, to achieve change, it can be worth risking some uncomfortable moments and challenging each other as to what is happening. Much will depend on the

| BOX 9.3 | *Some not uncommon hidden transactions that can occur in clinical supervision* |

Supervisor

- Adoption of a controlling or authoritative role with the supervisee, e.g. choosing to focus on poor practice or being unfairly critical
- Using humour to lessen the impact of a distressing situation rather than dealing with the real feelings of the supervisee
- Taking over the session to reduce emotion being shown by the supervisee because uncertain about their own reaction to the situation
- Diverting the conversation away from the supervisee's issue into an area the supervisor knows more about
- Wanting to maintain a popular image with supervisees by being their personal problem-solver (but by owning someone else's problems unwittingly adding to their own stress levels)
- Aware of being limited in facilitating reflective practice in others, so diverting the session into talking about their own previous experiences or holding a mini 'teaching' session
- Being 'far too busy' to attend their own 'supervisors' supervision' group because it might demonstrate to their peers how little they understand about supervision

Supervisee

- Not taking responsibility for the time spent during the session, e.g. avoiding issues, not using documentation, etc.
- Focusing on other people rather than themselves because worried that they might be being 'analysed', e.g. blaming the organisation for their own inadequacies
- Purposely elaborating on mistakes or misdemeanours in an attempt to minimise criticism by the supervisor
- Focusing throughout the session on why things have occurred rather than how they might be solved – talking is easier than actioning the solution in their practice
- Making out that everything is all right in clinical practice and that there is very little to discuss with the supervisor, therefore avoiding admitting any failings or weaknesses

Both supervisor and supervisee

- Making out that clinical supervision is useful and interesting, without any evidence to show that it is having any impact on organisational aims or patient/client care
- Pretending to know what clinical supervision is about, but not letting on to each other that they are not really very sure about what is expected of them – the workshops on clinical supervision were some months ago!
- Neither seeking out feedback on role performance for fear of not doing it right, as both are senior practitioners
- Finding that their initial enthusiasm for clinical supervision has waned, but neither wishing to rock the boat, as it is nice to have some regular time out away from clinical practice to talk about things
- Tending to agree with each other to avoid any unnecessary conflict, as clinical practice is stressful enough already

participants' understanding of clinical supervision and their willingness to challenge existing ways of communicating. Clinical supervision is an opportunity for both to learn about themselves, not just the supervisee!

Communication can be made easier right at the start of clinical supervision. The first session, as discussed in Chapter 5, should be an opportunity to make clear what each expects of the other and set boundaries in the form of a clinical supervision contract or agreement. Such an agreement should also include a date for a review, which would cover the unexpressed expectations or assumptions of both parties and how the supervision relationship is progressing (or not).

Transactional analysis is a useful tool with which to enhance communication in clinical supervision. The role of TA for communicating in nursing is explored in more depth by Ellis & Betts (1999). Effective clinical supervision is all about not just effective communication but particularly, as supervisors, being aware of the effect our preferred way of communicating has on others. Transactional analysis offers alternatives and the possibility not only of changing the way we interact with others in clinical supervision but also of acquiring a whole new set of communication skills for use both in practice and at home. To do this requires us to engage, for the most part, in Adult-to-Adult conversation. To distinguish Adult from Child or Parent communication, Stewart & Joines (1987, p. 14) suggest asking yourself: 'Was this behaviour, or thought, or feeling appropriate as a grown-up way of dealing with what was going on around me at that present moment? If the answer is "yes" then you are likely to be in Adult.'

Effective communication in clinical supervision requires both parties in the relationship to regularly consider this question in order to ensure that what is happening over the clinical supervision coffee table accurately reflects what is going on beneath it.

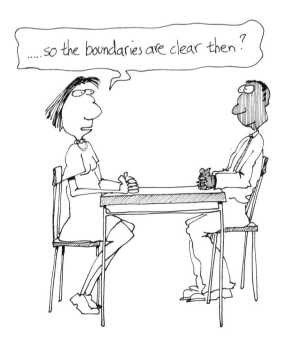

On reflection ... chapter summary

What are the key elements of this chapter?

- Being able to communicate effectively is an essential feature of a successful clinical supervision relationship
- Communication difficulties can be lessened by spending time in drawing up an explicit supervision contract or agreement that includes setting boundaries with each other and regular review dates
- Transactional analysis is useful for illuminating different communication behaviours between the supervisor and supervisee
- Transactional analysis offers different communication options and the possibility of changing existing patterns of communication
- Communication behaviours between the supervisor and supervisee can indicate the level of the clinical supervision relationship
- Hidden transactions are a maladaptive response to the stress of adopting new roles in clinical supervision
- Hidden transactions are an effective form of communicating in clinical supervision but when discovered can transform the relationship
- All supervisors should have a mechanism for discussing their supervisory practice with other supervisors

So what difference does this make to the way I am operating my clinical/ supervisory practice?

Now what actions will need to be taken as a result of my reflections?

REFERENCES

Bailey J, Baillie L 1996 Transactional Analysis: how to improve communication skills. Nursing Standard 35(10): 39–42

Berne E 1968 Games people play: the psychology of human relationships. Penguin Books, Harmondsworth

Dolley J, Davies C, Murray P 1998 Clinical supervision: a development pack for nurses (K509). Open University Press, Buckingham

Ewles L, Simnett I 1996 Promoting health: a practical guide, 3rd edn. Baillière Tindall, in association with the Royal College of Nursing, London

Ellis RB, Betts AM The Nurse as communicator Ch 17 pp 361–377. In: Kenworthy N,

Snowley G, Gilling C 1999 Common Foundation Studies in Nursing 2nd edn, Churchill Livingstone, Edinburgh

Inskipp F, Proctor B 1995 Cited in: Fowler J (ed) 1998 The handbook of clinical supervision – your questions answered. Quay Books, Salisbury, p 106

Kadushin A 1992 Supervision in social work, 3rd edn. Columbia University Press, New York

Stewart I, Joines V 1987 TA today: a new introduction to transactional analysis. Lifespace Publishing, Nottingham

10 From image to action: getting clinical supervision off the ground in the workplace

INTRODUCTION

Whether you are a staff nurse, a clinical manager, a potential clinical supervisor or a supervisee, there comes a point at which the image of what clinical supervision might look like in clinical practice needs to move from a vague theory into some form of workable reality. The early chapters of the book looked at some of the different agendas that need to be addressed before clinical supervision can be implemented in practice. Not least will be finding the time, in practice, to talk about practice on a regular uninterrupted basis.

One thing is for certain – it will not be possible to simply go it alone, or for one or two people to plan the system and impose it on the rest of the team (Clark et al 1998, p. 47). For a start, it requires management support for clinical supervision to be legitimised in practice and this will have to include finding the time and the financial resources. Other team members will require some information and discussion about what clinical supervision is. Some will need basic education on how to get the most from it.

This chapter will help you to approach setting up clinical supervision in your own area and highlight some of the factors that need to be considered before doing so. A parallel process to implementing clinical supervision in your own department or practice area will be to consider it also alongside managing any change in clinical practice.

A summary project plan is offered as a guide based on the author's ongoing experience of working with a number of NHS trusts and independent organisations to get the initiative off the ground. As Cutcliffe & Proctor (1998) wryly point out, there is no single method of implementing clinical supervision in nursing, but why should there be in such a diverse discipline as professional nursing? To be sustainable, clinical supervision will require practitioners working in their own specialism to contribute to how it should work in their practice arena. It is the underpinning principles of clinical supervision that are generalisable!

WHY CHANGE THE WAY YOU WORK ALREADY?

One of the overall themes of the book has been to suggest that, rather than adopt someone else's model of clinical supervision, efforts can be made to adapt what you have already. The chance meeting over coffee in the ward office or general practice coffee room with someone you trust or can confide in, or simply seeking out the 'parental figure' of your boss after a crisis has occurred may seem to you to be clinical supervision.

Now consider the following questions:

- Do you feel supported at work?
- Do you have a confidential forum where you can discuss your practice?
- Do you receive feedback about your clinical practice?
- Do you reflect upon your clinical practice and discuss these issues with an experienced practitioner?

Dooher et al (1998, p. 25) suggest if you answered 'No' to any of these questions it is time to seriously review or develop the system of clinical supervision in your practice area.

But finding regular and planned time to talk to somebody about your clinical practice, in practice time, rather than reacting to something after it has happened, is one of the biggest challenges in implementing clinical supervision. To achieve change in the way you are currently working requires thinking about the process of managing change as well as the process of implementing clinical supervision. As Smith (1995) rightly asserts: 'although clinical supervision may be needed in clinical practice it also has to be wanted by practitioners'.

While there is no professional argument about setting up clinical supervision, translating this into the everyday life of the unit is likely to be more difficult. So do not be surprised if your enthusiasm for clinical supervision, stemming from an introductory study day, workshops organised by your educational provider or reading around the subject, is not met with the same enthusiasm from practitioners who were working in the clinic in your absence and do not know as much about it as you.

PREPARING FOR THE CLINICAL SUPERVISION JOURNEY

Implementing any change in clinical practice can be likened to some of the exploits of the balloonists who tried to be the first to circumnavigate the globe.

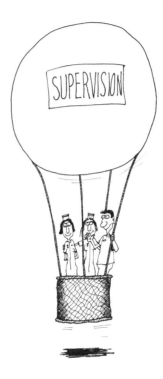

All the competitors want to be the first to get from point A to point B but their chances of getting there directly are remote, given the variable air currents, wind speeds, climate and technologies available. In reality, the intended direction of the balloonist is unlikely to be the actual route taken. What the balloonist requires is courage, skill and to be flexible enough to foresee the dangers and variables that exist, but at the same time not to lose sight of the ultimate objective, point B!

So it is with clinical supervision – you cannot embark on the journey without adequate backup and support, an assessment of the difficulties you are likely to face along the way and at least some idea of what to do if you get blown off course. Like the balloonist, the journey may be a bit turbulent and making the wrong decisions can bring you back to earth with a bump, as well as having some bruises to show for having engaged in the venture.

Think of some change that has taken place in your own practice area recently, e.g. the use of a new protocol or procedure – perhaps some new documentation has been introduced. Using the balloon analogy, reflect on how you and your colleagues managed to get from point A to point B.

What sorts of thing temporarily blew your unit off its main course?

Did you yourself have any specific role in manoeuvring the change back on course again?

To help with directing the clinical supervision balloon in your clinical practice area, it can be useful, prior to launch, to think of some of the things you will need to do to get off the ground successfully. Take-off is usually one of the scariest bits of the journey! It is useful to consider what you already do on a daily basis in looking after people – systematically work out a plan of action of what you intend to do. Steve Wright (1989, p. 7), a pioneer of many strategic changes in nursing practice, suggests that the implementing change is essentially a problem-solving exercise not dissimilar to the nursing process.

As an accountable practitioner you already plan your actions before implementing them and evaluate the success of the venture. So why not apply the same process on the clinical supervision journey? Central to introducing supervision into clinical practice will be the strategies employed by you as an individual practitioner, collectively as a staff group and the organisation you work for.

ASSESSING WHAT NEEDS TO HAPPEN ON THE WARD/IN THE HEALTH CENTRE

The journey starts by assuming that either you have read something about clinical supervision in a journal or that you have just returned from a study day about clinical supervision armed with information and a number of different ideas. An interested colleague or manager may well ask you what the study day was about, and you cite a definition of clinical supervision taken from the original *Vision for the Future* document issued by the Department of Health: 'Clinical supervision ... is a term used to describe a formal process of professional support and learning which enables individual practitioners to develop knowledge and competence, assume responsibility for their own practice and enhance consumer protection and safety of care in complex situations' (Department of Health 1993).

Although offering the 'what' and 'how' of clinical supervision, such definitions are intended as starting points and can sometimes appear to be 'ideal types' that get lost when comparing them to the realities of your own clinical area. It is more useful to get a discussion going in order to achieve some consensus with work-based colleagues about what clinical supervision might look like in your area of practice.

The UCL Hospitals NHS Trust, in London, offered the following position statement after extensively collaborating with clinical practitioners and South Bank University to reach consensus on the 'what' and 'how' of clinical supervision:

> Clinical supervision is perceived to benefit the quality of patient care, the organisation and particularly the individual nurse because it gives a regular opportunity to share and discuss clinical experiences in a constructive manner. It also enables nurses to be innovative in a supportive environment. It is a formal relationship, with the process and ground rules agreed at the start, which enables nurses to regularly reflect on their practice with another, or other experienced nurses, in order to learn from experience and improve their competence and can be undertaken in a variety of ways, ranging from a group, to one-to-one supervision (UCL Hospitals NHS Trust 1997).

This type of definition really gets to the heart of doing clinical supervision in practice, as well as describing the 'how' and 'what' of clinical supervision. It is also backed up by the organisation itself. To make real sense, however, further translation and ownership will be required from the staff in the unit. But before some consensus statement or definition can be made for your own clinical area, you will first of all need to know what your colleagues know about clinical supervision. This will mean not keeping to yourself the information you have read or brought back from the study day but sharing it around. A good way to do this is to flag up clinical supervision as a discussion item in a ward meeting and share your information to gauge some initial reactions from your colleagues. Designate an area, e.g. a filing cabinet drawer, to start collecting information on clinical supervision that can be referred to by other staff, including those who are not there when you are. Why not also designate one or two people to be the resource or link people about clinical supervision?

The first stage of launching clinical supervision, then, is to generate and disseminate information about the possibilities that exist for the practice area. The aim is to raise awareness and stimulate discussion around the ward while at the same time preparing yourself and colleagues to address the specifics of how you intend going about clinical supervision in your unit. In essence, you are assessing the needs of the unit before formally planning how to go about clinical supervision. Some considerations for doing this are listed in Box 10.1.

BOX 10.1	*Assessing what needs to happen to launch clinical supervision in your practice area*

- General interest by one or two staff members, e.g. through reading or attendance at a workshop
- Organise a way you and your interested colleagues can collect data and information about clinical supervision
- Find an area in the unit where information can be collected and consulted
- Talk to your educational provider, or contact people you already know who are involved in clinical supervision, to get some ideas
- Fix a workable time to review the relevant data as a staff group
- Set some regular meetings with representatives of the unit to identify some of the probable challenges implementing it will involve, e.g.:

  - what the staff group understand the term 'clinical supervision' to mean
  - what the purpose of doing it is
  - what is needed in terms of training and education
  - how you intend to find the time
  - who will be the supervisors and supervisees
  - what the most likely mode of doing it is
  - where it should happen

- Decide on a lead person who will have responsibility for overseeing the process within the unit
- Draw up your own unit position statement as a staff team on what clinical supervision is and is not and let each staff member have a copy of it

Although you might think that this part of implementation is too time-consuming, it is useful to be clear not only about the direction in which you intend to travel but also about what form other people on the unit think clinical supervision should take. This will save you time when confronted by the inevitable challenges that might blow you off course later on in the project. Having a person from outside to guide your preliminary meetings is useful to ensure that the limited time is used effectively and to mediate any differences of opinion. Obviously, it is essential that all meetings are documented or recorded in some way, as they will be taking place during working hours. This will also provide useful data for any write-up that you may wish to do later. The use of Action Learning Sets focussing on these issues in setting up clinical supervision is more fully described in Royal College of Nursing Institute (1999) and West Midlands Clinical Supervision Learning Set (1998)

At this point it is useful to be aware that clinical supervision will involve the allocation of planned time during working hours for the activity. This will inevitably mean that there will be cost implications as well as logistical difficulties in trying to cover busy workloads. You cannot attempt to set up a clinical supervision system in the workplace without consulting your line manager first. There are five good reasons for this (Box 10.2).

BOX 10.2	Five reasons why you need to consult your line manager about your interest in clinical supervision

- Your line manager needs to endorse the activity, as it involves allocation of resources – it is no good staff feeling supported at work if there are no nurses in the clinic to look after patients
- Managers are very likely to have heard about clinical supervision and, unknown to you, may already be helping with strategic plans for the initiative within the organisation
- You can formally declare your own interest in clinical supervision and this may lead to working with others within your organisation who are similarly interested
- Managers can support you in managing the necessary organisational changes as they are likely be more experienced and are involved in this type of activity on a daily basis
- Managers will know through their own networks who you can liaise with and how you can learn more, e.g. allowing a visit to a neighbouring trust to see how clinical supervision is operating already or funding your attendance at relevant study days

Another assessment that is extremely useful if you are really serious about the success of the venture is to consider the forces that will be at work during the project. Doing so before you launch the initiative will ensure that all staff are aware of the influences that will ultimately determine whether clinical supervision in your workplace succeeds or founders.

FORCES THAT AFFECT PLANS TO IMPLEMENT CLINICAL SUPERVISION

If we once again use the analogy of the clinical supervision balloon discussed earlier, we can assume that getting from point A to point B will be eventful, and is unlikely to take a direct route. The route is more likely to be as outlined in Figure 10.1.

| Figure 10.1 | *A likely route for implementing clinical supervision in practice* |

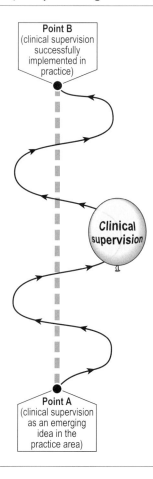

The broken line represents a hypothetical direct route from point A to point B. It is helpful to think about the 'flying time' the unit intends to allocate to the project (e.g. 6 months), and whether this takes into account being blown off course, and also what to do in the event of a crash landing.

There will be a number of different forces that will enable you to reach your desired goal of implementing clinical supervision – motivated staff, enthusiasm, etc. – but ranged against them will be opposing forces preventing you from achieving it – e.g. finding the time for clinical supervision during a busy shift.

Bowman (1990, p. 104) describes these forces as pushing forces (those that will keep you airborne along your intended route) and resisting forces (those that will blow you off your intended route). If the pushing forces are stronger than the resisting forces you are likely to be moving in the right direction. If not, your implementation plan needs to be adjusted. Therefore, in the assessment and planning stages of setting up clinical supervision you may wish to do your own ward 'force field analysis'.

Consider your own clinical area in relation to Figure 10.2, which depicts an imaginary ward that has already implemented clinical supervision over a 6-month period. The central broken line represents the route (and timeframe) they originally intended to take. See how the resisting forces move you away from your intended route and can extend the journey time, while the pushing forces keep you close to getting where you want to go.

Can you, or preferably your staff group, think of some likely pushing forces in your area other than those illustrated?

What other resisting forces might your unit face?

MINIMISING AND MAXIMISING THE FORCES THAT EXIST

Having considered some of the pushing and resisting forces in your practice area, to keep up the momentum and continue in the right direction Bowman (1990, p. 104) suggests that three things need to happen, which can also form a structure for your ongoing discussions:

- strengthen the pushing forces
- weaken the resisting forces
- add some new pushing forces to the ones you already have.

Some common pushing forces in implementing clinical supervision are summarised in Box 10.3, along with some additional ways of keeping the ward close to its intended direction.

Inevitably, as with any intended change to practice, there will be resistance. Broadly speaking, resistance is a way of saying 'No!' to change. But when handled sensitively, because you had planned for it, resistance can also make a valuable contribution to the implementation of clinical supervision.

In order to weaken any forces resisting your implementation of clinical supervision, it is useful to understand why they are occurring, rather than reacting in a hostile or defensive way to them.

Look at the following reasons why clinical colleagues are likely to be resistant to clinical supervision. How can you change these opinions? In reality, you will not have to deal with as many all at the same time, but they are drawn from a collection of clinical supervision workshops for various nursing directorates.

'I don't know much about it.'

'We're too busy to start something like that.'

'The term "supervision" sounds like another managerial tool to beat me up with.'

'I can't see how it's supposed to benefit me.'

'Clinical what? It's just another buzzword that if left alone for long enough will go away.'

'I wouldn't trust him/her as a supervisor.'

'I had an appraisal last year.'

'There's no need for me to have it – I'm one of the most senior staff here.'

'I'm retiring in two years and I'm not changing my way of working to please you or anybody else!'

'We're doing it already anyway.'

'Oh, that's for students – not experienced staff like most of us here!'

Within the paradox that change is the only thing likely to remain constant in nursing lies the irony that the object of certain nurses' resistance – clinical supervision – could provide some relief from the pressures that such changes have created (Wilkin et al 1997). Perhaps, as McCallion & Baxter (1995) point out, the resistance to change has something to do with the way clinical supervision is presented to practitioners in the field – being interpreted, for example, as a management monitoring exercise dreamed up to check up on practitioners, or being based on the ideas of a couple of staff rather than a collective effort.

In many respects, the fact that you can elicit this type of response to clinical supervision in your work area is in itself helpful. Now there is an array of identifiable issues that upset practitioners about clinical supervision. Many of the responses reveal that practitioners feel they have little power or control over events. It is interesting to speculate how a clinical supervisor might respond to these if presented with them in a group or individual situation.

My own responses to the reactions set out above would be to try to make the practitioner believe that they did have some control over how clinical supervision unfolds in their work situation. The first step in confronting issues that supervisees bring to clinical supervision is often to simply help them identify and acknowledge their concerns, in order that they can then begin to move forward. After that, clinical supervision will be directed towards exploring different options and agreeing some form of feasible actions that will help the supervisee with their concerns.

'It's all right for you to say that,' I can imagine some readers of this book saying, 'you don't have to set it up on my ward!' Perhaps another potential solution might work better for you – eliciting the help of someone who does not work in your clinical area. Strategies for weakening some of the resisting forces you may experience in implementing clinical supervision are summarised in Box 10.4.

In addition to strengthening the pushing forces and weakening the resisting forces, to continue the clinical supervision momentum and get extra movement

Figure 10.2 *Some imaginary pushing and resisting forces in implementing clinical supervision in clinical practice*

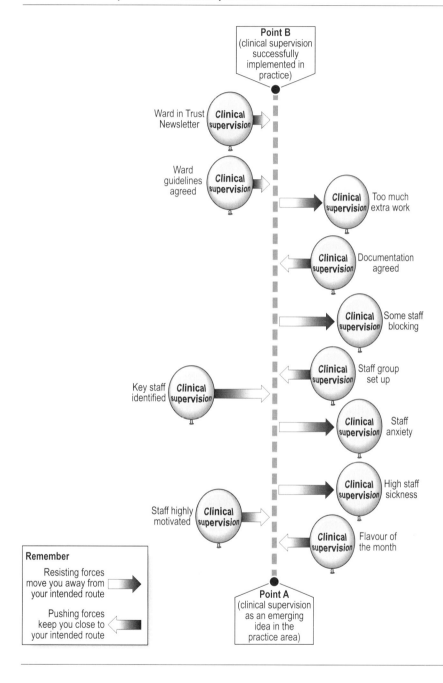

on the unit your group might like to think about adding some new pushing forces to the ones you already have (Box 10.5).

Perhaps now, as a highly motivated individual nurse interested in setting up clinical supervision in your ward or health centre, you are beginning to realise

BOX 10.3	Strengthening the pushing forces for implementing clinical supervision

Pushing forces	Strengthening pushing forces
Staff motivated at start of pilot project	Allow one or two interested members of staff to organise the gathering of information and find a central area to store the material Keep key members of staff in touch with other areas involved in the initiative to compare ideas and learn from each other Use incentives such as attendance at relevant courses or meetings, supporting where necessary time for organising material
Planning meetings sanctioned by ward manager	Ask the staff to come up with ways they think they can manage to attend, given existing workloads Suggest a workable time frame for the staff to work towards and set dates, times and venues of meetings beforehand Provide the resources to release staff to attend the meetings Lobby the ward manager to ensure clinical supervision is included in the Annual Trust Business Plan
Key members of staff identified	Ensure key members of staff represent the whole unit including those who are on rotational night duty or on holiday Lobby the ward manager for one staff member to represent your clinical area on any steering group your organisation may have formed Work out some sort of rota so that all unit staff can eventually attend clinical supervision workshops
Staff planning group or Action Learning Set organised	Consider whether you wish to share the 'chairing' of meetings or to get the help of an outside facilitator, e.g. a practice development nurse Ask for feedback from or minutes of the meetings without necessarily controlling it yourself Aim for a space during meetings to consider how to action emerging ideas Document what happens Set out some structure of how you intend using the time together (Box 10.1) Consider the likely areas of resistance to clinical supervision in the unit and how you intend managing these Think before you start about how you intend to monitor the effectiveness of clinical supervision on the ward/in the health centre

BOX 10.3 Cont.	*Strengthening the pushing forces for implementing clinical supervision*
Pushing forces	**Strengthening pushing forces**
Preliminary documentation produced	Assign some time to read the literature on documentation to save reinventing the wheel Liaise directly with people outside your unit to see what is being produced elsewhere Ensure that your documentation broadly embodies any organisational policy being produced simultaneously
Ward/practice guidelines agreed	Start off by trying to write a ward/practice statement on clinical supervision that most staff endorse Lobby your manager to make a case for additional funding where necessary to support your guidelines e.g. if clinical supervision is to take place on a one-to-one basis each month Include the guidelines in any induction package for new staff Make the training department aware of your guidelines – perhaps one of your staff members could be included in any talk being given to new staff on clinical supervision
Publication of the initiative in the organisation's newsletter	Rake out some of the documentation you have kept that might help you reflect on the journey you have all been on Lobby senior managers to make sure your achievements are recorded in any annual review of the organisation Invite interested outside parties to visit your ward or unit Try to get an interested party to help you write up some of your findings in setting up the initiative for a national journal – it will contribute to our knowledge about clinical supervision and put your ward efforts on the map! Consider setting up a formal or informal project to monitor the life and effectiveness of clinical supervision over the next year in your ward

the enormity of it all, and how to be successful requires a planned and systematic team effort that must also include managerial support. One of the best ways of finding out more about clinical supervision is to experience it first-hand yourself. You may even wish to investigate how you can contribute to the setting up of clinical supervision in your own area by obtaining your own clinical supervision, where this is possible. If it is not, you will have to resort to moving things forward by talking to your team group and getting your manager on board.

If, as Wilkin et al (1997) suggest, clinical supervision is about offering staff the opportunity to reflect on and develop clinical practice, you are already well on the way to developing this culture in your own clinical environment. You must have begun meeting regularly as a group to get this far. The important thing is for the meetings not just to be 'talking shops' but to agree to convert some of the talking into action within an agreed timeframe, in other words, become Action Learning Sets!

BOX 10.4	*Weakening the forces resisting the implementation of clinical supervision*

Resisting forces	Weakening resisting forces
Lack of information	Only think about implementing clinical supervision after adequate discussion of what it means to individuals and the clinical environment Encourage selected staff to attend in-house workshops, roadshows or similar events and disseminate information to colleagues Aim for one or two members of staff to co-ordinate the collection and sharing of information for the ward/health centre Consider some staff members networking with other departments or practices to bring in outside information Arrange a clinical supervision awareness meeting hosted by someone who has been through the process of setting it up elsewhere
Staff mistrust of each other	This needs to be communicated to the line manager, not just in order to implement clinical supervision but to increase staff harmony Consider having regular ward meetings facilitated by an outside person to find out why mistrust exists Consider incorporating a choice of supervisor into the local guidelines rather than allocating them
Not enough time/time spent in clinical supervision adversely affecting clinical care	Consider whether this is a blocking activity or whether reorganisation of nursing work is required Ask staff to come up with their own ways in which clinical supervision time might be found The ward/practice manager might carry out an audit of nursing work to analyse more fully how time is being spent The ward/practice manager could lobby support for extra funding and resources for clinical supervision
Clinical supervision not seen as a high priority	Discuss whether existing support structures are adequate Discuss what benefits implementing clinical supervision might have for the delivery of care Give information on professional, managerial and educational agendas for implementing clinical supervision
Supervision viewed as a management tool, e.g. appraisal	As above (lack of information) In order to work, clinical supervision requires support from management but the local organisation should come from within the practitioner staff group
Senior staff not considered to need it –staff cynicism about yet another buzzword	As above (lack of information) Clinical supervision is not mandatory and it may be worth investing the resources in newer and more motivated staff used to the concept of reflective practice and lifelong learning Manager and willing senior staff should act as supervisee role models before expecting the rest of the staff to participate

BOX 10.5	*Ways of increasing the pushing forces on the unit to increase the momentum of clinical supervision*

- Don't be too over ambitious: you have to learn to fly the balloon before you can attempt to circumnavigate the world!

- Identify individual staff responsible for carrying out one or more of the actions arising from your team discussions

- Ensure there is an adequate way that all staff on rotational nights, days off, etc. can access what is going on with the project ... not just the staff who happened to be working on the day any new directions are decided

- Chart your progress for disseminating lessons learned from the project

- Work closely with the ward/practice manager and supply adequate data and information from staff meetings to assist in his/her lobbying for increasing staff resources and support to carry out your specific requirements

- Never be afraid to go to other people with more experience than yourself in clinical supervision – even neighbouring organisations or departments such as local education providers, professional bodies, authors of journal articles

- Set deadlines to monitor progress at the beginning of the project and undertake corrective actions if being blown off course

- Consider what as a staff group you regard as successful implementation of clinical supervision and incorporate this into any subsequent formal evaluation or audit

Two principles for effective clinical supervision are that you must set a date some time in advance to critically review together what has been happening and whether changes must be made and that you must, at the end of each session, agree on action to follow up what you have been discussing. Both of these principles apply to the implementation of clinical supervision. By setting up the initiative you are experiencing clinical supervision already ... but perhaps were not aware of it!

SPECIFIC CONSIDERATIONS WHEN IMPLEMENTING CLINICAL SUPERVISION

For clinical supervision to become embedded into the culture of clinical practice it has to be owned by the practitioners themselves and adequately supported by the organisation. Many of the opposing forces emerge from lack of information and misunderstanding. In addition to this, if clinical supervision is not adequately resourced and time is not dedicated to the management of the project, the venture will begin to collapse.

In my opinion, it can sometimes be useful for the staff team to be honest enough to say at the outset to the clinical manager: 'At this point, with our existing resources, we are not able to give our best attention to getting clinical supervision started.' This will prevent you from setting off in a piecemeal way only to see the initiative fall flat on its face. Dolley et al (1998, p. 146) reassure practitioners that, despite the high profile of clinical supervision, implementing

BOX 10.6	*Essential issues for clinical staff to address in order to implement clinical supervision*

- How will we find the time?
- How shall we go about it?
- How will we know if investing in it will benefit ourselves, the organisation and our patients?
- What will be the ground rules for it?
- Where can it take place?
- Who should have it?

- Who will be the supervisors?
- What sort of training will be required?
- How much is this all going to cost?

it on the ward or in the health centre will initially be experimental and the ways that it is carried out will vary. The important thing is that you get going with something most of you have agreed upon – finding 'the right way' of doing clinical supervision is a goal that is still up for grabs and it might be your own unit that sets the standard for everyone else. There are, however, essential elements in the practice of clinical supervision about which decisions will have to be made by the staff; these are summarised in Box 10.6. Some of these elements may already be contained within your organisation's policy or protocols for clinical supervision.

If your own unit is still trying to mobilise support and resources, it can be helpful to set up some transitional arrangement such as a regular facilitated staff group or Action Learning Set once a month with the aim of reflecting on whatever the group feels is appropriate. At the same time, one or two other committed staff members might wish to be 'seconded' to help an adjoining area set up their own clinical supervision initiative, in order to learn from their mistakes! In tandem with this, as has already been suggested, any staff wishing to take up clinical supervision with the pool of supervisors that already exists in the organisation should be encouraged to do so and report back to the staff group.

Two very practical issues for clinical environments considering clinical supervision are:

- affording the time
- finding a suitable environment.

Affording the time

It is interesting to speculate whether readers considering implementing clinical supervision view it as an outlay to the organisation in time or money, or an investment. Can your organisation afford not to support their practitioners through the promotion of clinical supervision while at the same time presenting to prospective employees a caring ethos towards not only their patients but also their best resources – the human ones? Perhaps the cost of not having clinical supervision will not be in monetary terms only?

But what about the cost of having clinical supervision? Butterworth et al (1997, p. 16), in their multisite study, set minimum requirements for clinical supervision time of 45 minutes every 4 weeks and the range was between 25 minutes and 1.5 hours every 2 weeks. Group supervision was reported to take longer, lasting between 1.5 and 2 hours.

The advantages and disadvantages of different types of supervisory mode require discussion by the ward group – some may only wish to participate in the relative safety of an individual session with a supervisor, while others may prefer to work in groups. While the relative merits of the different modes of supervision are discussed elsewhere (Hawkins & Shohet 1994, Brown & Bourne 1996, Bond & Holland 1998, Butterworth et al 1998, Dolley et al 1998, West Midland Clinical Supervision Action Learning Set 1998, Royal College of Nursing Institute 1999), it is not difficult to cost clinical supervision in terms of how many staff times how often and for how long. What is more difficult is finding the time to do it.

Can you remember when you last had an uninterrupted dinner break in the staff restaurant (or out of the health centre) *or* two separate coffee breaks of about 20 minutes during a shift?

If your answer to the above was 'No', what would you do if you received an internal memo from the chief executive's office stating that as from tomorrow you were to have regular meals of the above duration to comply with a European Health and Safety at Work Directive he/she had received – *how would you then find the time?*

If your answer was 'Yes', would you be prepared to trade in the above on one occasion per month if you were allowed to take in your refreshments to the supervision room?

While the abovementioned European directive is fictitious, it is interesting to speculate how you would find the time, if it was not. Perhaps, as it was deemed to be for the good of your own health and came from the highest levels of the organisation you would more readily comply. This is one way, albeit perhaps unrealistic, of getting yourself along to clinical supervision because a) it has been officially legitimised by the organisation or b) it is personal to you as a practitioner.

Peter Nicklin, an independent health consultant in a national conference on clinical supervision in Coventry, asked for a show of hands to the question 'How many of those here present have worked the equivalent of 1 hour over the time they were contracted for in clinical practice?'(Nicklin 1997). In my estimation (I was in the conference room) almost three-quarters of the audience raised their hands. According to his research findings, Nicklin (1998) reckons that nurses are contributing, or are owed, £50 million in unpaid overtime – the estimated cost of implementing clinical supervision across the UK!

Finding a suitable environment

A questionnaire about clinical supervision sent to all trust nurse executives in England and Scotland highlighted the lack of suitable venues in many NHS trust sites (Bishop 1998, p. 32). Does this apply to where you intend to do clinical supervision?

Dolley et al (1998, p. 48) suggest that the immediate environment of the supervision venue will offer the following, which will usually be under the control of the practitioner:

- privacy
- comfortable seating
- an appropriate room
- easy access
- acceptable levels of background noise
- access to some refreshment
- facilities for any special needs.

Where in your place of work do you think that the foregoing conditions might be found?

Would you accept anything less than this for engaging in clinical supervision, or would it mean having to leave the unit?

Should the clinical supervision environment feature when you are agreeing rules and setting boundaries in the first session?

If the environment was required not for clinical supervision but for interviewing a relative, where would that be?

PULLING IT ALL TOGETHER: A 'CARE PLAN' FOR SETTING UP CLINICAL SUPERVISION IN PRACTICE

Much of this chapter has been involved with the importance of assessing and planning what needs to happen before the implementation of clinical supervision – before the balloon goes up on the unit. If you were looking after a patient/client, the way you would go about this would be to allocate a primary nurse or key worker and organise care using a problem-solving approach. So why not instead write your own 'care plan' for the unit to give the clinical supervision balloon some direction (Figure 10.3).

The notion of a 'care plan' is not a patronising one. There are four reasons for this:

- It is better to use a familiar tool to carry out complex work

- The nursing process is cited as a useful way of managing change

- Clinical supervision is essentially a professional support mechanism for staff on the unit. In other words, systematically planning what you intend doing is an act of caring for one another that will then impact on the way you care for others

- It not only offers a framework to give you some direction and manageable, bite-sized chunks of implementation to be getting on with, but also reminds you that in addition you must consider how you will know if it is working or not.

Figure 10.3 A 'care plan' for clinical supervision (continued on next page)

Assessing – issues to consider for getting supervision started	Planning – how we intend to go about it as a staff group, including who will be responsible for what	Implementing – what we intend to happen clinically and by when
1. Not sure who knows what on the ward about clinical supervision	Delegate two staff members to organise a questionnaire for all staff to establish a baseline for the project	*Short-term goal:* No decisions to be made about implementing clinical supervision until all qualified staff have been consulted
2. Collect some data and information about clinical supervision	Gather the information: literature search, college librarian, contact professional bodies, liaise with relevant staff in the organisation/mental health unit, network with others outside organisation	*Short-term goals:* Two staff volunteers to co-ordinate activity and report to the first meeting of the transitional group Ask for assistance of link tutor and practice development nurse Charge nurse to set aside office space for information
3. Working out what resources will be needed to establish the project	Involve the clinical manager to advise on resources and what is happening elsewhere Document everything as it happens for manager and for any subsequent evaluation *First phase:* Set up a named transitional group arrangement *Second phase:* Continue with or set up a new project group or action learning set	*Short-term goals:* Obtain commitment of clinical manager to advise on the project and assist with resources Forward minutes and documentation of transitional group for discussion with charge nurse during management supervision (weekly) *Longer-term goals:* 10 fortnightly meetings to get some feedback from representative staff group about clinical supervision Force field analysis and focused discussion on implementing clinical supervision on the unit
4. Establishing how we can all communicate with one another about clinical supervision	Consider getting an external person from the college or practice development nurse to help with the first-phase group	*Short-term goal:* Liaison staff to be appointed (volunteered!)

Assessing – issues to consider for getting supervision started	Planning – how we intend to go about it as a staff group, including who will be responsible for what	Implementing – what we intend to happen clinically and by when
5. Getting staff interested in the project while doing the work	Some introductory clinical supervision study days available on current educational contract	*Longer-term goal:* Allow some key staff to get experience of clinical supervision in the interim to cascade down to other staff
6. Working out the length of time it will take to get started, including a launch date to work towards	Arrange for feedback and advice from clinical supervision data collection jointly with project group	*Intended timing:* Information gathering and reporting – 4 weeks Transitional group – 10 fortnightly meetings (5 months) Education programme to be arranged Launch on unit – 6 months
7. Working out how staff would prefer to organise the mode of delivery of clinical supervision	Dependent on staff feedback and information-gathering exercise, including staff questionnaire	Following on from information gathering and reporting – 4 weeks
8. Working out who should give and receive clinical supervision, e.g. support workers?	With present resources initially only trained staff, but will review after first evaluation	*Longer-term goal:* Clinical supervision to be included in the induction programme for all new staff
9. Making clear to staff their roles and responsibilities in clinical supervision	Arrange for education provider used by the organisation to devise an educational programme for ward staff, e.g. supervisor and supervisee workshops 3 months before launch – no gaps between education and launch date! Seek out clarification within the organisation of how supervisors will get supervision	*Longer-term goal:* Liaise with any organisational steering group about policy and standards/protocol and devise own position statement on clinical supervision for the unit, as well as documentation, e.g. local guidelines, contracts, supervision records, audit material *Longer-term goal:* Get any of our 'trained' supervisors on the organisational database
10. Assessing the effectiveness of clinical supervision	Will seek advice while transition group operating	*Longer-term goal:* Implement and monitor clinical supervision on the unit over 6 months and 1 year
Other things to include as they arise:	Review care plan at each fortnightly meeting	Named person at each meeting to take minutes and update care plan

Keep the care plan in a drawer in the ward office.

The 'care plan' is not intended to be prescriptive but to give an overview of how different your project can look on paper when it is systematically reviewed and key issues or questions are addressed. This is different from simply chatting in the hectic atmosphere of the unit about what you might do. Like reflective practice, which demands not only thinking but action, so does the nursing process or 'care plan'. Regularly writing up what goes on will be helpful for any planned evaluation you may do, and is covered more fully in Chapter 11. Although there have been some indicators in this chapter as to the organisational implications of implementing clinical supervision, the main aim was to focus on some common ward activities.

You may also wish to refer to Kohner (1994), Brocklehurst (1996), Sams (1997), Bishop (1998), Bond & Holland (1998), Rafferty et al (1998) West Midlands Clinical Supervision Action Learning Set (1998), Royal College of Nursing Institute (1999) and your own specialist journals for more specific information on organisational implementation of clinical supervision. It can also be helpful to network directly with the UKCC and with lead nurses (often in practice development departments) who have first-hand experience of the challenges associated with implementing clinical supervision across whole organisations. The most rewarding aspect of your efforts can be reviewing what sort of potential differences regular clinical supervision could make to your clinical area. This is covered in Chapter 11.

On reflection ... chapter summary

What are the key elements of this chapter?

- Implementing clinical supervision is a ward team event that requires managerial support to do so successfully
- The first stage of implementation will be gathering information and discussing as a team what your vision of clinical supervision should look like on the unit
- There is no preferred or single method of implementing clinical supervision
- The way you initially set out to implement clinical supervision will very likely be different from the route taken
- The process of change is not dissimilar to the nursing process that nurses are already familiar with
- Having an external person to facilitate your ideas in the unit can be useful
- Determining beforehand what sorts of forces are at play in implementing clinical supervision can help you to avoid problems later in the project
- Clinical supervision can provide some relief from the constant changes that practitioners face
- Set up transitional groups or action learning sets prior to implementing clinical supervision

So what difference does this make to the way I am operating my clinical/ supervisory practice?

Now what actions will need to be taken as a result of my reflections?

REFERENCES

Bishop V 1998 (ed) Clinical supervision in practice – some questions, answers and guidelines. Macmillan/Nursing Times Research Publications, London

Bond M, Holland S 1998 Skills of clinical supervision for nurses. Open University Press, Buckingham

Bowman C 1990 The essence of strategic management. Prentice Hall, Englewood Cliffs, NJ

Brocklehurst N 1996 Clinical supervision in the West Midlands: a survey of NHS Trusts. Health Services Management Centre, University of Birmingham, Birmingham

Brown A, Bourne I 1996 The social work supervisor. Open University Press, Buckingham

Butterworth T, Carson J, White E, Jeacock A, Clements A, Bishop V 1997 It is good to talk. An evaluation study in England and Scotland. School of Nursing, Midwifery and Health Visiting, University of Manchester, Manchester

Butterworth T, Faugier J, Burnard P 1998 Clinical supervision and mentorship in nursing, 2nd edn. Stanley Thornes, Cheltenham

Clark A, Dooher J, Fowler J, Philips A, North R, Wells A 1998 Implementing clinical supervision. In: Fowler J (ed) The handbook of clinical supervision – your questions answered. Quay Books, Salisbury, ch 2, p 47

Cutcliffe JR, Proctor B 1998 An alternative training approach to clinical supervision: 1. British Journal of Nursing 7(5): 280–285

Department of Health 1993 Vision for the future: report of the Chief Nursing Officer. HMSO, London

Dolley J, Davies C, Murray P 1998 Clinical supervision: a development pack for nurses (K509). Open University Press, Buckingham

Dooher J, Fowler J, Philips A, North R, Wells A 1998 Demystifying clinical supervision. In: Fowler J (ed) The handbook of clinical supervision – your questions answered. Quay Books, Salisbury, ch 1, p 25

Hawkins P, Shohet R 1994 Supervision in the helping professions. Open University Press, Milton Keynes

Kohner N 1994 Clinical supervision in practice. King's Fund Centre, London

McCallion H, Baxter T 1995 Clinical supervision – how it works in the real world. Nursing Management 1(9): 20–21

Nicklin P 1997 Research – it's good to talk! Joint conference paper (presented with Professor Tony Butterworth) at the Whatever Happened to Clinical Supervision? Conference at the Post House Hotel, Coventry, UK, 12 November 1997, organised by PNK Associates and the Nursing Times

Nicklin P 1998 Clinical supervision: what is it? In: Bishop V (ed) Clinical supervision in practice – some questions, answers and guidelines. Macmillan/Nursing Times Research Publications, London, ch 1, p 14

Rafferty M, Jenkins E, Parke S 1998 Clinical supervision: what's happening in practice? A report submitted to the Clinical Effectiveness Support Unit (Wales). School of Health Science, University of Wales, Swansea

Royal College of Nursing Institute 1999 Realising clinical effectiveness and clinical governance through clinical supervision a distance learning pack. Radcliffe Medical Press, Oxon, UK

Sams D 1997 Clinical supervision: an evaluation of the implementation process within a community trust. Unpublished BSc(Hons) dissertation, South Bank University, London

Smith JP 1995 Conference report: Clinical Supervision: conference organized by the National Health Service Executive at the National Motorcycle Museum, Solihull, 29 November 1994. Journal of Advanced Nursing (21): 1029–1031

UCL Hospitals NHS Trust 1997 Guidelines for clinical supervision at UCL hospitals. UCL Hospitals NHS Trust, London

West Midlands Clinical Supervision Learning Set 1998 Clinical supervision: getting it right in your organisation A critical guide to good practice. West Midlands Clinical Supervision Learning Set, University of Birmingham, UK

Wilkin P, Bowers L, Monk J 1997 Clinical supervision: managing the resistance. Nursing Times 19(93): 48–49

Wright SG 1989 Changing nursing practice. Edward Arnold, London

11 Monitoring the effectiveness of clinical supervision in practice: is the truth already out there?

INTRODUCTION

Perhaps this final chapter should have been the first, as monitoring the effectiveness of clinical supervision should be one of the first things to consider in practice, rather than being tagged on as an optional extra at the end of a project. But to begin clinical supervision with the end in mind is extremely difficult, as the concept is not yet a feature of everyday nursing practice. Therefore any potential benefits or outcomes for practitioners and their patients will be understandably somewhat tentative.

Even the UKCC (1996) leaves evaluation until the end of its position statement on clinical supervision, asserting that there is currently a lack of information on clinical supervision in practice. It sensibly suggests that local evaluation systems be developed to assess how clinical supervision influences care, practice standards and the service.

For those of you just commencing or thinking about clinical supervision in practice an analogy comes to mind – whether to invest in digital television. Some people will already have jumped in and bought the system (along with all the potential teething problems), while others prefer to see first what the impact will be before setting up their own system. The latter group have the luxury of not only being able to invest in a system that has come down drastically in price, but will also have more knowledge of the benefits and outcomes of owning it.

It is important to remember that reflecting on and documenting what is happening in clinical supervision is an important part of the implementation process and will contribute to evaluating its effectiveness both for individual supervisees and for the unit as a whole. This chapter offers those considering putting a system of clinical supervision into practice a means of monitoring its success and a reassurance that the lessons learned, if disseminated to others, will help to contribute to the national landscape of clinical supervision in nursing.

THE NEED TO MONITOR THE EFFECTIVENESS OF CLINICAL SUPERVISION IN PRACTICE

As you are probably already aware, the 'doing' of clinical supervision in practice is not an exact science. There always seems to be something new to read or talk about. The diversity of settings in which clinical supervision occurs and the potential benefits of regularly engaging in it make monitoring extremely challenging.

There are at least five good reasons for monitoring the effectiveness of clinical supervision in practice (Box 11.1).

BOX 11.1	*Five reasons for monitoring the effectiveness of clinical supervision in practice*

- There is currently a lack of information on the benefits and outcomes of having clinical supervision in practice
- Employers have invested in clinical supervision largely on the assumption that it will be advantageous in clinical practice and will therefore need to be convinced that further investment is warranted
- In quality-conscious healthcare settings clinical supervision will not be sustainable without some form of measurable outcome monitoring its effectiveness or lack of it
- To supply evidence for the effectiveness of clinical supervision in practice in order to strengthen the case for employing organisations to fully support the initiative by incorporating it into the annual business plan
- To provide an opportunity for the whole ward/health centre team to make a contribution to the development of clinical supervision knowledge in nursing practice rather than accepting someone else's ideas about what it is

The UKCC accepts that there is currently a lack of information on the benefits and outcomes of having clinical supervision in practice, yet many healthcare organisations have actively encouraged clinical areas to get started. This has formed the basis for some authors (Nicklin 1995, Wolsey & Leach 1997, Dimond 1998a, 1998b, Rogers 1998, Yegdich 1998, 1999) to challenge the efficacy of widespread implementation of clinical supervision in nursing practice with so little research-based evidence to support it.

If you have already begun clinical supervision in your own practice area, your team will need to consider assessing how clinical supervision is impacting on care delivery and the service. Many employers, perhaps your own, have invested in clinical supervision as what Butterworth (1998, p. 229) calls 'acts of faith' in the advantages that clinical supervision is felt to offer. It does not take much working out to assume that such 'acts of faith' by employers will reach a point where decisions will have to be made about whether to continue with clinical supervision or not. This decision will be based on whether clinical supervision is viewed as being effective, not only for practitioners engaging in it but, more importantly, for any impact on patient care as a whole.

Question your manager about what *they* understand about clinical supervision in practice and compare this to the reasons *you* see as important for engaging in it.

If you haven't already been sent to read up the practice guidelines on clinical supervision as a response to this question by your manager, compare how the guidelines really reflect the views of yourself and your manager.

What contradictions, if any, emerge as a result of this exercise? It may form the basis for any monitoring of clinical supervision you are planning as a ward/unit team if you know beforehand what your organisation expects from clinical supervision and what is actually happening.

Inevitably in quality-conscious healthcare settings, clinical supervision will not be sustainable without some form of measurable outcome. Implementing clinical supervision is in effect a microcosm of the managerial and economic climate in healthcare, which has radically changed in the last decade (Woods 1998, p. 40). Therefore all the emphasis currently placed on increased productivity, through-put, endless demands with scarce resources and the demand for quality in health-care by a new administration (Department of Health 1998, Brocklehurst & Walshe 1999) will also apply to clinical supervision. Interestingly, Dooher et al (1998, p. 22) and Fish & Twinn (1997, p. 89) imply that the clinical supervisor might already fulfil a quality assurance function by ensuring that professional standards in the nurse–patient relationship are maintained.

Butterworth et al (1997), in their government-sponsored multisite evaluation of clinical supervision, begin to offer empirical evidence that clinical supervision and mentorship schemes protect as well as support clinical staff in practice, but recommend that staff must be given adequate time and preparation to adapt to the additional roles and responsibilities. While it could be argued that the selected sites were motivated by being involved in the project, as well as by being given the financial support to evaluate the effectiveness of clinical supervision, only two of the 23 sites had actually incorporated it into their NHS Trust annual business plans.

Therefore, putting systems in place to monitor the effectiveness of clinical supervision will ensure that, while still viewed as an 'act of faith', there is documented evidence to lobby for its inclusion in a more fully resourced annual business plan. Many non-nurse managers may not be familiar with Key Statement 4 of the UKCC position statement on clinical supervision (1996), which states: 'Every practitioner should have access to clinical supervision'.

Without lobbying for a firm organisational commitment to clinical supervision by putting forward ways in which its effectiveness can be monitored, it is unlikely that enough resources will be made available to give it a fair trial in clinical practice.

Giving a firm commitment to the organisation not only to engage as practitioners in clinical supervision but also to document what is happening in your unit as a whole will also allow you develop ways of doing clinical supervision that suit your local needs. In this way, all practitioners involved in clinical supervision can contribute to shaping how it develops. By doing this, you will also be developing 'clinical supervision knowledge' that is specific to your own specialist practice. You could also enlist the help of your practice development team, clinical nurse specialist, audit department or educational provider to devise ways in which this could happen.

INDIVIDUAL REFLECTION ON EFFECTIVE CLINICAL SUPERVISION IN PRACTICE

The different aspects of clinical supervision offered in the previous chapters of this book can assist you in drawing together some monitoring signposts for your own practice area.

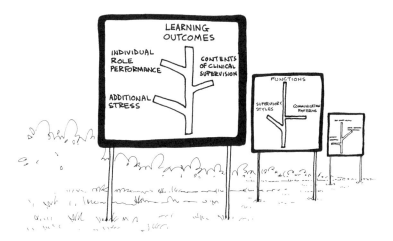

The sorts of thing that can be monitored and have previously been covered are:

- How clinical supervision differs from similar activities used in practice
- The initial contents of clinical supervision contracts and why they change (if at all), e.g. changing the supervisor, whether supervisee-led, etc.
- The learning outcomes of education-provider clinical supervision packages against the uptake of clinical supervision in practice
- What method of doing clinical supervision works in your area and why
- What individual functions of clinical supervision can be observed in practitioners engaging in clinical supervision, e.g. more accountable, increased learning, feeling more supported
- The individual role performance of the supervisee in clinical supervision as reported by the supervisor
- The individual role performance of the supervisor in clinical supervision as reported by the supervisee
- Any reported additional distress caused to the supervisor by facilitating clinical supervision in others

- The different supervisory styles and approaches used, as reported by either party in supervision
- What communication patterns appear to enhance the sessions
- Ways in which the supervisee reports that engaging in clinical supervision improves care delivery
- How the initial strategy for implementation in the clinical area is evolving
- How all the above could be documented or collected without breaching confidentiality.

Breaking down clinical supervision into its different component parts is easier than thinking of it as a whole and how it can be monitored for effectiveness. One of the obvious things to do is to keep some record or documentation of what happens in clinical supervision, rather than having to remember something about it when asked.

In many ways, this is exactly parallel to the process of clinical supervision itself. Initially, a supervisee can be overwhelmed by the number of things to talk about in such a short space of time. But, as the sessions progress, the supervisee learns to focus on particular issues to deal with and improve upon in clinical practice. Any monitoring of the effectiveness of clinical supervision should ideally be based in the supervisees' personal experience, as it is they who understand how effective or ineffective it really is.

Clinical supervision is a method of formalised reflection on practice. The What? model of structured reflection, alluded to in an earlier chapter, is a useful structure to get individuals started in monitoring what constitutes effective or ineffective clinical supervision (Figure 11.1) If you recall, to be reflective requires you to actively process your experiences and convert them into some workable form of action, and is different from simply thinking about practice.

Purposeful reflection (as if in a session) on what is happening can help to identify the potential markers of effective or ineffective clinical supervision in practice. In essence, then, the truth of effective clinical supervision practice may already be embedded in practice – it simply needs to be identified. Let us assume that in your own practice area you have recently implemented clinical supervision and that your ward manager has set practitioners a target of 6 months to review its effectiveness. On the basis of the earlier reflective activity, some potential markers to measure against might be:

- an uninterrupted session
- not feeling guilty about leaving the clinical work
- completing writing up what happened in time for the next session
- being able to choose one's clinical supervisor
- the use of an audio cassette by the supervisee to help them remember what went on and allow some continuity
- the session led by what the supervisee, not the supervisor, determines as important practice issues
- the availability of refreshments
- the supervisor not discussing what went on in the session with others in the health centre/on the ward.

It has been suggested that one of the most important people to consider in monitoring the effectiveness of clinical supervision is the supervisee. Look at Figure 11.1 and, using the trigger questions in Box 11.2 to help you, if necessary, reflect upon two accounts of your personal experience of clinical supervision that focus on:

- A meaningful clinical supervision session for me was…
- A not-so-meaningful clinical supervision session for me was…

When you compare the two accounts, why were they so different despite the fact that you may have been describing sessions facilitated by the same supervisor?

What can you or your supervisor do in future sessions to limit a not-so-meaningful session and enhance more meaningful sessions?

If you have not engaged in clinical supervision yet, what in your opinion might constitute a meaningful or not-so-meaningful clinical supervision session, based on what you have read or heard? I would suggest that much of what goes on in clinical supervision has yet to be fully identified and articulated. Perhaps many individuals, having taken the plunge and engaging in regular clinical supervision, now have what they consider to be effective clinical supervision.

Figure 11.1   *The revised WHAT? model of structured reflection and its relationship in monitoring the effectiveness of clinical supervision in practice*

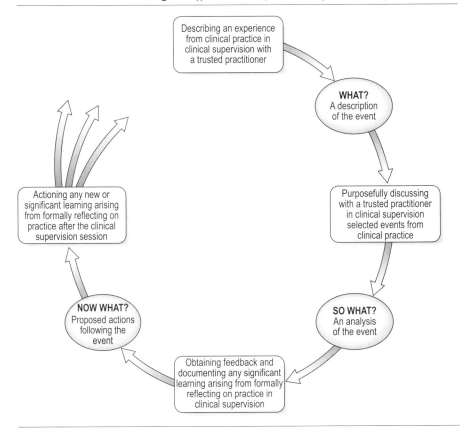

| BOX 11.2 | *The revised WHAT? model of structured reflection and associated trigger questions* |

1. **A** *description* **of the event**
   WHAT? trigger questions:
   - is the purpose of returning to this situation?
   - happened?
   - did I see/do?
   - was my reaction to it?
   - did other people do that were involved in this?

2. **An** *analysis* **of the event**
   SO WHAT? trigger questions:
   - How did I feel at the time of the event?
   - Were those feelings I had any different from other people who were also involved at the time?
   - Are my feelings now, after the event, any different from what I experienced at the time?
   - Do I still feel troubled? If so, in what way?
   - What were the effects of what I did (or did not do)?
   - What positive aspects now emerge for me from the event?
   - What have I noticed about my behaviour in practice by taking a more measured look at it?
   - What observations does any person helping me to reflect on my practice make about the way I acted at the time?

3. **Proposed** *actions following* **the event**
   NOW WHAT? trigger questions:
   - What are the implications for me and others in clinical practice based on what I have described and analysed?
   - What difference does it make if I choose to do nothing?
   - Where can I get more information to face a similar situation again?
   - How can I modify my practice if a similar situation was to happen again?
   - What help do I need to help me 'action' the results of my reflections?
   - Which aspect should be tackled first?
   - How will I notice that I am any different in clinical practice?
   - What is the main learning that I take from reflecting on my practice in this way?

You can probably think of many others, based on your own personal accounts. Although such things might seem obvious and trivial, it is possible to measure all of them and this can lay the foundation for monitoring your clinical supervision scheme more formally.

IDENTIFYING PERFORMANCE INDICATORS IN CLINICAL PRACTICE FROM THE FUNCTIONS OF CLINICAL SUPERVISION

While documenting individual attributes and characteristics of what goes on in clinical supervision is important, other performance indicators can also be used. Butterworth & Bishop (1994, pp. 42–44) suggest that it is possible to audit clinical supervision through existing reporting mechanisms (Box 11. 3).

BOX 11.3	*Existing reporting mechanisms that can be used to audit clinical supervision*
	■ Clinical audit
	■ Rates of sickness and absence
	■ Staff satisfaction scales
	■ Number of patients' complaints
	■ Retention and recruitment of staff
	■ Critical incident maps
	■ Stress and burnout assessment tools
	■ Staff health questionnaires
	■ Trust-wide educational audit
	■ Individual performance review
	■ Live supervision recorded on video or audio tape
	■ *Post hoc* analysis of audio or video tape recordings
	■ Live or *post hoc* analysis of supervision observation notes

Others that could also be included are:

■ patient satisfaction surveys

■ increased compliance with PREP requirements, e.g. those currently on paid study leave, professional portfolio completion, attendance at study days

■ observing any increased innovation/practice development

■ an increasing number of supervisors being included on any published database or lists

■ collating numbers of staff currently engaged in clinical supervision

■ greater awareness of individual risk management, e.g. increased practitioner accountability

■ improved record-keeping.

The amount of indirect data available to link to clinical supervision in the practice area is formidable but I would suggest, dovetails into also collating evidence for clinical governance that is already happening in practice. More obvious are any formal or informal research projects being undertaken within the organisation associated with what is happening in clinical supervision. With so much potential data to collate, it can be difficult to know where to start.

The composite elements of clinical supervision described in an earlier chapter (Proctor 1986) are helpful to remind practitioners what the purpose of clinical supervision is. Each of the broad functions of clinical supervision, while overlapping, can offer a framework in which to place the most appropriate monitoring tools (Figure 11.2).

Figure 11.2   *The three functions of Proctor's interactive model of supervision*

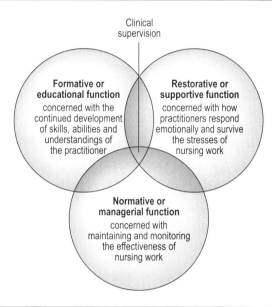

Monitoring the effectiveness of clinical supervision using these functions separately may lead to a narrow, or even biased view of what is happening in clinical supervision practice. For instance, monitoring the support functions of clinical supervision only, will fail to address other potentially effective elements supervision offers the practitioner, such as improved learning or increased managerial awareness, that impact on service delivery. When used together they can offer a more detailed picture of what happens in clinical supervision (Bowles & Young 1999).

Look at the three functions of Proctor's interactive model of supervision in Figure 11.2. Which previously identified performance indicators of clinical supervision (Box 11.3) equate to Proctor's functions of supervision?

So far this chapter has tended to look at the different markers and ways that the effectiveness of clinical supervision can be monitored retrospectively – in other words, after clinical supervision is up and running the individual experience of supervision or the implementation of the initiative as a whole is assessed. But it is also possible (with the consent of all parties), to monitor effectiveness during 'live' episodes of clinical supervision, with the aid of an observer or audio-visual aids. This method is particularly useful to research what is happening as it happens, and a useful tool for clinical supervision training.

Course participants on the ENB RO1 (Clinical Supervision Skills for Supervisors) course at South Bank University, London, devise their own tool for obtaining feedback on supervisory performance as part of their course requirements (Figure 11.3). In reality, evaluating the effectiveness of clinical supervision is likely to be a trust-wide venture or involve a whole unit.

It can save a lot of time to decide at the outset to work towards getting a consensus statement on what people in the unit agree is an acceptable way of doing clinical supervision. For those yet to set it up in practice, agreeing evaluative markers is part of the implementation process discussed in Chapter 10. Many practitioners will bring in to such discussions their personal expertise of writing practice statements and setting standards.

Setting practice standards in clinical supervision based on known or likely performance indicators will help to make it more visible to those questioning its efficacy. It also creates a practice-specific audit tool that involves all practitioners in devising ways of measuring the effectiveness of clinical supervision.

A PROVISIONAL PROFESSIONAL STANDARD FOR CLINICAL SUPERVISION IN THE WORKPLACE

Clinical audit is not an unfamiliar term in healthcare. It means improving clinical effectiveness by giving practitioners an opportunity to obtain feedback on what is being done in practice (*Nursing Times* & NHS Executive 1998, p. 13). Not at all unlike clinical supervision! The process involves practitioners measuring their practices against previously agreed standards and modifying it where indicated as a result of the audit (NHS Executive 1996). This same process can be applied when working as a group to agree practice guidelines in clinical supervision.

To be measurable in practice, setting standards for clinical supervision must first be agreed by practitioners who will be involved in it. The steps in setting standards for clinical supervision adapted from Blackie (1998, p. 208) are outlined in Box 11. 4.

BOX 11.4	*The steps in setting standards for clinical supervision*

- Select aspects of clinical supervision practice
- Select performance indicators of quality clinical supervision practice
- Identify criteria and a level of performance in clinical supervision using an agreed standard-setting framework
- Devise and agree written standards for each of the criteria set on level of performance in clinical supervision practice using a measurable instrument, e.g. ideal, average, minimum, unacceptable, etc.

As with clinical audit, the emphasis is on continual improvement by making modifications to the standards as you go along, based on what is found to be happening in clinical supervision practice. The Donabedian structure, process, outcome, method of dynamic standard setting, pioneered by the Royal College of Nursing (1990), will now be a familiar audit tool to most practitioners.

| Figure 11.3 | *A supervisory feedback tool devised by ENB R01 participants to monitor the effectiveness of a clinical supervision session* |

Faculty of Health

ENB R01
CLINICAL SUPERVISION FOR CLINICAL SUPERVISORS
EVALUATION SHEET FOR OBSERVER

	EVIDENT		COMMENTS
	YES	NO	
INTRODUCTION			
a) Punctuality			
b) Greetings (warm & friendly)			
c) Agenda - Issues from last session - New issue/s for this session			
d) Venue Conducive, comfort, privacy, distraction			
e) Boundaries set			
STRUCTURE			
a) Length - 1 hour max.			
b) Boundaries maintained			
SUPERVISORY FUNCTIONS			
1. Reflective Learning			
2. Accountability in Practice			
3. Supportive			
OUTCOMES			
a) Achievement of goals			
b) Was supervisee happy with outcome?			
c) Was supervisee left supported?			
d) Was there an action plan drawn up?			
e) Was supervisor given feedback?			

JD/JK/ENB R01-Cohort 02/99
Joy, Brenda, Heather, Pam, Paul, Mariola, Jonathan, Pauline

Devising and writing standards in clinical supervision practice using a structure–process–outcome model allows each element to be examined independently, not just the outcome that was aimed at. Fowler (1998, p. 57) reminds us that, when writing standards in clinical supervision, we should be SMART about it and that statements should be:

- Specific
- Measurable
- Achievable
- Realistic
- Timed.

A simplified structure–process–outcome approach to standard setting in clinical supervision for your own unit would be to address the questions listed in Box 11.5. They will require some baseline knowledge of what clinical supervision is, in order to be able to set the standards you wish to achieve in practice.

BOX 11.5	*A simplified structure–process–outcome approach to standard setting in clinical supervision*

- What is it that you want to achieve, as a group of practitioners, with your clinical supervision standard? (**The outcome**)
- How do you intend, as a group of practitioners, to achieve the desired clinical supervision standard? (**The process**)
- What sorts of thing will you need, as a group of practitioners, to help you reach your clinical supervision standard? (**The structure**)

Select **one** baseline performance indicator for clinical supervision that you think your unit would view as important. Look at the earlier part of the chapter to remind you of the possibilities.
  Using the structure–process–outcome format, try to write a single SMART statement for standards in clinical supervision practice. You may wish to compare your own with mine (Box 11.6).

Considering the use of standard setting when implementing clinical supervision has a number of advantages and disadvantages (Box 11.7) and was central to the development of clinical supervision by practitioners in Wales.

The development of clinical supervision in Wales has been markedly influenced by the drive for it to also be clinically effective in practice (Welsh Office 1997). Although perhaps not dissimilar to the aspirations of your own organisation, measuring the effectiveness of clinical supervision in mid- and west Wales used a previously developed provisional standard in clinical supervision adopting the structure–process–outcome approach to standard setting (Rafferty et al 1998).

Developed by practitioners already experienced in clinical supervision, in conjunction with the University of Wales (School of Health Science Swansea), the provisional standard uses as its standard statement: 'Professional supervisory relationships will utilise contracts based on the following structure to

BOX 11.6	*An example of single standard statement for clinical supervision practice using the structure–process–outcome format*

A standard statement in clinical supervision practice

Prior to engaging in clinical supervision, all supervisees on the unit should have some idea of what to expect in the first session.

Structure	Process	Outcome
The content of the 3-hour education package needs to be agreed by the Directorate but must include the need for establishing written contracts between the supervisor and supervisee. The dates, times and venues of the package need to be agreed and made known to all line managers in the Directorate. Financial arrangements need to be agreed between the organisation and the education provider. The package must be continually monitored and updated where necessary, based on written evaluations by those attending. A 6-monthly summative report must be submitted to the Directorate by the course co-ordinator, including any recommendations.	Any practitioner seeking clinical supervision for the first time must inform the nurse in charge so arrangements can be made for them to attend a supervisee workshop. Accurate attendance records must be forwarded to the Directorate on completion of each course by the course co-ordinator. Each participant will be required to complete a written evaluation at the end of each workshop. An accurate 'live' clinical supervisor database must be maintained by the practice development nurse and made available to all new supervisees on request. The Directorate will provide a broad clinical supervision contract for use in the workshop that may be adapted to meet the needs of the practitioner in clinical supervision in agreement with their supervisor.	Each practitioner on the unit intending to engage in clinical supervision will first attend a 3-hour supervisee workshop run within the Directorate.

create and maintain opportunities for support and learning that promotes accountability, harm prevention, clinical development and emotional competence' (Rafferty et al 1998, p. 78).

Further standard statements are then made for each of Proctor's functions of supervision, previously discussed, which are labelled Professional support (Box 11.8), Learning (Box 11.9). and Accountability (Box 11.10).

BOX 11.7	*Some advantages and disadvantages of standard setting when implementing clinical supervision*

Advantages

Provides a forum for implementing quality clinical supervision

Encourages the development of knowledge because of the need for practitioners to be aware of key issues relating to the implementation of clinical supervision

All practitioners can be involved in agreeing the content

Specific elements of clinical supervision related to local needs are addressed

The resources required to achieve the desired outcomes are more easily identifiable within the structure and process

It provides data to argue the case for adequate resources before full implementation

Local standard setting can inform more centralised practice guidelines

Differences between what is wanted from clinical supervision and what is actually achieved in practice can be identified and changes made

Provision of data on the effectiveness of clinical supervision locally can contribute to any setting of national standards

Disadvantages

Time consuming

More paperwork

Alterations to the standard need to be communicated to all those using it

Initial disputes in devising an agreed content

After completion may simply be filed away until a few days before audit

Looking at each of the standard statements that contribute to the landscape of clinical supervision in Wales, how might the structures seen as important for each of Proctor's functions of supervision be translated into your own practice area?

Perhaps in your own area of practice, 'environment' might not be considered to be important as part of Professional Support, whereas finding the time would be. Bear in mind that the provisional standard is intended to cover different institutions over a large geographical area.

Would your own organisation benefit from attempting to break down each element of Proctor's functions of supervision in order to obtain a broad measure of the effectiveness of clinical supervision? How can standards in clinical supervision be set from existing practice guidelines that may have been adapted from a single centralised organisational policy to suit the myriad local needs of, for instance, mental health, district nursing or acute adult nursing?

Although evaluation is often the last thing to do in a project, for clinical supervision to continue it is crucial to develop criteria, or markers, in tandem with any implementation. Unfortunately, this book falls into the same trap. While there must be some sympathy for those who state that clinical supervision should not be implemented without evidence supporting its efficacy in

BOX 11.8	Professional support standard statement: 'The necessary pre-conditions for professional support relate to time, environment and relationship issues'. (Reproduced with permission from Rafferty et al 1998, p. 78).	
Structure	**Process**	**Outcome**
Time	Rational judgements are made about the necessary time to meet emotional and developmental tasks which take account of supervisor, supervisee and organisational requirements	It is demonstrated that time is available for supervision in line with rational decisions leading to the determination of models of good practice
Environment	Arrangements are made to ensure that the environment will be conducive to privacy, comfort and the prevention of inappropriate distraction	Individuals confirm the environment is suitable, or otherwise, for supervision and behaviours (including posture and verbal reports) are adopted which maintain or lead to a change of accommodation
Relationship	Attention is paid to creating an egalitarian relationship which acknowledges power differences by attending to issues of honesty, choice, mutual respect, sensitivity, tolerance and the potential to use uncertainty and vulnerability productively	Statements about emotions and congruent behaviours from supervisees confirm that acceptable and/or unacceptable growth-focused relationship values are evident in the supervisory process and appropriate action is taken

practice, the same argument could be applied to reflective practice. At least such authors are increasing the profile of clinical supervision by generating some badly needed critical comment.

Like reflective practice, clinical supervision requires an innovative approach to justify its efficacy. The uncertainty that clinical supervision brings with it, despite not being empirically based at present, is that it remains, in most cases, practice-led. Monitoring its effectiveness is not a sterile academic exercise, it is crucial for clinical supervision to be sustained in practice.

The tools for monitoring that effectiveness, which have been the subject of this chapter, are not unfamiliar to practitioners. But unless we begin to think of clinical supervision with some sort of end in mind – e.g. setting evaluative criteria or standards – then it may well disappear into the limbo of good ideas that did not materialise in nursing ... or be made compulsory instead.

The clinical governance agenda is not dissimilar to the principles of clinical supervision and may help the formal legitimisation of it. Both aim to support and develop staff by providing the opportunity to adopt good practice and

BOX 11.9	Learning standard statement: 'Facilitating practice learning involves supervisory interventions which focus upon practice and relevant knowledge and skills'. (Reproduced with permission from Rafferty et al 1998, p. 79).

Structure	Process	Outcome
Focus	The focus of supervision is the supervisees' expression of their professional practice experience (including the experience of supervision) and reflection upon its meanings	Accounts about supervision provided by the supervisee and supervisor identify that practice and its professional and personal meaning is the focus
Knowledge	Meaning arises from the study of supervisees' explanations of practice in terms of human dynamics with the understanding that this can always be developed by searching for what is known, not known and necessary to know, to enhance professional practice	Accounts about supervision provided by the supervisee and supervisor acknowledge degrees of professional and emotional competence and identify the dynamic nature of learning
Interventions	Interventions affirm appropriate practice, personal support and professional esteem and the search for developmentally achievable professional challenges	Feedback about supervision provided by the supervisee and supervisor includes reports about increased professional well-being and plans of action to utilise professional competence and meet learning needs

BOX 11.10	Accountability standard statement: 'Organisational and personal accountability is enabled through the utilisation of information which allows professional judgements to be made about competence'. (Reproduced with permission from Rafferty et al 1998, p. 80).

Structure	Process	Outcome
Organisational support	The organisation provides the necessary will and resources to enable supervisees and supervisors to respectively receive or offer appropriate supervision	Organisational monitoring identifies the patterns of supervisory practice and their match with strategic direction and resources
Recording	Supervisees, supervisors and the organisation responsibly negotiate models of supervisee-held records which specify minimum content and the conditions for access designed to acknowledge good practice and limit harm	Both good and potentially harmful practices are identified and effectively responded to as part of the evaluative process
Competency	Competent supervisory practice requires the use of appropriate authority and the recognition of personal and professional boundaries.	Supervisors' supervision ensures that the exercise of authority and maintenance of personal and professional boundaries is appropriate.

learn from experience, as well as addressing poor clinical performance (Royal College of Nursing 1998, Department of Health 1999). The Bristol Inquiry is only at the halfway stage (Davidson 1999) and will undoubtedly influence the implementation of clinical governance and clinical supervision as a mechanism for the delivery of effective nursing care. Depending on the recommendations of the Bristol Inquiry, clinical supervision may even be forced on to practitioners. Even the UKCC's position statement on clinical supervision (UKCC 1996) left the door ajar for reviewing it as a statutory requirement, as it is in midwifery. Perhaps the cost of compulsory clinical supervision in practice would at least be a fully resourced and clinically effective system of supervision in our quality-conscious healthcare organisations. The jury is still out on clinical supervision, and it is practitioners alone who are charged with issuing the only correct verdict – a non-mandatory system of clinical supervision regulated and monitored for its effectiveness by those same practitioners who engage in it. After all, between them they have more than enough expertise.

On reflection ... chapter summary

What are the key elements of this chapter?

- Monitoring the effectiveness of clinical supervision should be one of the first, not last things to consider in any project

- There is currently a lack of information on the effectiveness of clinical supervision in practice

- Documenting what happens in clinical supervision is an important part of monitoring its effectiveness

- Organisational decisions to continue clinical supervision will be based on the impact clinical supervision is having on patient care delivery

- In quality conscious healthcare settings clinical supervision will not be sustainable without some form of measurable outcomes regarding its effectiveness in practice and links in to the clinical governance agenda

- The clinical supervisor may have a quality assurance function

- Firmer organisational commitment to clinical supervision can be achieved by devising systems in practice to monitor its effectiveness

- Setting practice standards helps to make clinical supervision more visible to those questioning its efficacy

- Setting standards in clinical supervision will contribute to measuring its effectiveness and ensure quality supervisory practice

So what difference does this make to the way I am operating my clinical/ supervisory practice?

Now what actions will need to be taken as a result of my reflections?

REFERENCES

Blackie C 1998 Quality. In: Blackie C (ed) Community health care nursing. Churchill Livingstone, Edinburgh, ch 11, p 208

Bowles N, Young C 1999 An evaluative study of clinical supervision based on Proctor's three function interactive model. Journal of Advanced Nursing 30 (4): 958–964

Brocklehurst N, Walshe K 1999 Quality and the new NHS. Nursing Standard 13(51): 46–53

Butterworth T 1998 Evaluation research in clinical supervision: a case example. In: Butterworth T, Faugier J, Burnard P (eds) Clinical supervision and mentorship in nursing, 2nd edn. Stanley Thornes, Cheltenham, ch, 15 p 229

Butterworth T, Bishop V (eds) 1994 Proceedings of the Clinical Supervision Conference held at the National Motorcycle Museum, Birmingham, 29 November. NHS Executive, London

Butterworth T, Carson J, White E, Jeacock A, Clements A, Bishop V (1997) It is good to talk. An evaluation study in England and Scotland. School of Nursing, Midwifery and Health Visiting, University of Manchester, Manchester

Davidson L (1999) Iron fist, kid gloves. Health Service Journal (July): 24–27

Department of Health 1998 A first class service – quality in the new NHS. 13175 NUR 13k 1P (June). HMSO, London

Department of Health 1999 Clinical governance: quality in the new NHS. Health Service Circular (HSC) 1999/065. Department of Health, Leeds

Dimond B 1998a Legal aspects of clinical supervision 1: Employer vs employee. British Journal of Nursing 7(7): 393–395

Dimond B 1998b Legal aspects of clinical supervision 2: Professional accountability. British Journal of Nursing 7(8): 487–489

Dooher J, Fowler J, Philips A, North R, Wells A 1998 Demystifying clinical supervision. In: Fowler J (ed) The handbook of clinical supervision – your questions answered. Quay Books, Salisbury, ch 1, p 22

Fish D, Twinn S 1997 Quality clinical supervision in the health care professions – principled approaches to practice. Butterworth-Heinemann, London

Fowler J (ed) 1998 The handbook of clinical supervision – your questions answered. Quay Books, Salisbury

NHS Executive 1996 Clinical audit in the NHS. Using clinical audit in the NHS: a position statement. NHS Executive, Leeds

Nicklin P 1995 Super supervision. Nursing Management 2(5): 24–25

Nursing Times & NHS Executive 1998 Clinical effectiveness for nurses, midwives and health visitors (supplement, July). Nursing Times & EMAP Healthcare, London

Proctor B 1986 Supervision: a co-operative exercise in accountability. In: Marken M, Payne M (eds) Enabling and ensuring – supervision in practice. National Youth Bureau, Council for Education and Training in Youth and Community Work, Leicester, pp 21–34

Rafferty M, Jenkins E, Parke S 1998 Clinical supervision: what's happening in practice? A report submitted to the Clinical Effectiveness Support Unit (Wales). School of Health Science, University of Wales, Swansea

Rogers P 1998 Hype that is hard to swallow (opinion). Mental Health Practice 1(10): 18

Royal College of Nursing 1990 Dynamic standard setting system. RCN, London

Royal College of Nursing 1998 Guidance for nurses on clinical governance. Order no. 000 941. RCN, London

UKCC 1996 Position statement on clinical supervision for nursing and health visiting. United Kingdom Central Council for Nursing, Midwifery and Health Visiting, London

Welsh Office 1997 Welsh Nursing and Midwifery Committee plenary: Clinical Supervision and Clinical Effectiveness. HMSO, London

Wolsey P, Leach L 1997 Clinical Supervision: a hornet's nest or honey pot? Nursing Times 93(44): 24–29

Woods D 1998 The therapeutic use of self. In: Butterworth T, Faugier J, Burnard P (eds) Clinical supervision and mentorship in nursing, 2nd edn. Stanley Thornes, Cheltenham, ch 3, p 40

Yegdich T 1998 How not to do clinical supervision in nursing. Journal of Advanced Nursing 28(1): 193–202

Yegdich T 1999 Clinical supervision and managerial supervision: some historical and conceptual considerations. Journal of Advanced Nursing 30(5): 1195–1204

Conclusion

So I come to the end of this book on the practice of clinical supervision. I sincerely believe that normalising critical reflection on practice, through clinical supervision, will really make a difference to those diverse nursing worlds that make up the discipline of nursing. Clinical supervision has so many possibilities for nurse practitioners, their organisations and, most importantly, the people we are charged with caring for. But the process cannot be rushed, despite the need to be more accountable in practice through clinical governance and clinical effectiveness schemes. The work ethic of clinical practice will not change, but there must also be a genuine concern for the personal health of the workforce from within the healthcare factory.

Such possibilities can only be realised by practitioners letting go a little bit and seeking out some regular practice space. This is one of the first challenges – valuing yourself enough as a practitioner to be able to stop and critically reflect on your practice, with others who are very likely to have similar concerns. This may well mean looking at existing methods of work and making a conscious decision to change them. In order to care for others, it is important that individual practitioners look after themselves, otherwise they will find themselves too much in need of support to be able to give any.

Implementing clinical supervision offers an opportunity to become reacquainted with team members, as well as forging new alliances in the struggle to make it a practice reality. Practitioners, not theorists, are deciding how best to organise and implement clinical supervision, and rightly so. The challenge is in 'rethinking' oneself in practice, which has for so long been dominated by non-practitioners telling practitioners what and how to nurse. This is a part of the heritage of nursing that is now being challenged and is at last being 'unlearned' by means of critical reflection on practice. Clinical supervision offers a lifeline for concerned practitioners to safely explore how the practice of nursing can be enhanced and made more effective.

As we enter the new millennium there is a new awakening in nursing practice. This has been brought about by a critical mass of practitioners who, when critically reflecting on their practice, are dissatisfied with the way they work. For individuals used to reacting to crisis situations, clinical supervision also offers an opportunity to be more proactive about practice – but with others to support the new ideas and thinking, not alone. Often, to get real change means weathering conflicts that will arise as practice evolves. The challenge is for organisations to become more transparent and actively help groups of concerned practitioners to achieve change by working together. Supporting clinical supervision is also supporting political activism in nursing – the evolution of which is not so surprising, now the roots of nurse education are firmly embedded in higher education.

In an earlier chapter, I suggested a 'Doomsday scenario' for clinical supervision if practitioners were unwilling, or not supported, to develop clinical supervision as an optional activity. In many ways, because there is so much expectation of clinical supervision in practice, not having it at all now seems unthinkable. It is essential that the critical mass of staff continues to lobby for clinical supervision schemes that are voluntary, and focuses on the personal and professional development of practitioners, in the belief that this will enhance practice. Making clinical supervision mandatory for practitioners might be useful in the short term to ensure that staff take it up. While this might guarantee some sort of efficient return on investment, it will not guarantee effectiveness. Similarly, the investment must also extend to ensuring that new clinical supervisors are able to obtain their own supervision to support their new role and are not simply viewed as icing on the clinical supervision cake.

Clinical supervision supports the clinical governance view that there is no endpoint to learning in nursing. But are 'new' practitioners, who will be aware of the traditional supervision continuum in nursing (e.g. supervised practice/preceptorship) also made aware of the nature of clinical supervision after qualification? Such new practitioners also need some form of preparation for clinical supervision, despite the idea that they are already reflective practitioners! And what of the preparation of supervisees and supervisors? It would be helpful if there was some baseline knowledge about the necessary education and training for both!

Although we have reached the end of this journey, I suspect that clinical supervision will continually evolve in nursing, albeit slowly. Already by the time of its completion, this book will require updating as the search for quality clinical care steps up a gear with the implementation of clinical governance alongside clinical supervision. As part of the evolving process of clinical supervision, you, the reader, are invited to offer your comments, thoughts and ideas about the content of this book and, more importantly, to contribute to the knowledge of clinical supervision in nursing. You can continue this dialogue by e-mail on johnd@tlc-uk.com or by contacting John Driscoll at Transformational Learning, Consultants Park Lodge, Waldingfield Road, Gallows Hill, Sudbury, Suffolk CO10 6QS, UK.

Index